The Posture of
Meditation

Will Johnson

The Posture of Meditation

*A Practical Manual
for Meditators of All Traditions*

SHAMBHALA

BOSTON & LONDON

1996

Shambhala Publications, Inc.
Horticultural Hall
300 Massachusetts Avenue
Boston, MA 02115
www.shambhala.com

9   8   7   6   5

Printed in Canada

♾ This edition is printed on acid-free paper that meets the
American National Standards Institute Z39.48 Standard.

Distributed in the United States by Random House, Inc.,
and in Canada by Random House of Canada Ltd

Library of Congress Cataloging-in-Publication Data
Johnson, Will, 1946–
The posture of meditation: a practical manual for
meditators of all traditions/by Will Johnson.
p.   cm.
ISBN 1-57062-232-9
1. Meditation.   I. Title.
BL624.2.J65   1996   96-7535
158'.12—dc20   CIP

This book is dedicated to all those people who have had the good fortune to bring a sitting meditation practice into their lives, in hopes that the information here may further assist and support them in their practice.

Contents

Acknowledgments

I WOULD LIKE to express my thanks and appreciation to all my teachers of sitting meditation: Koon Kum Heng, Tarthang Tulku, Ruth Denison, Hari Das Baba, Yogi Bhajan, Jack Kornfield, Joseph Goldstein, S. N. Goenka, and Namkhai Norbu. Special thanks and acknowledgment must go to Ida Rolf, who led me to understand that the harmonizing of the energy field of the body with the gravitational field of the earth is a prerequisite for spiritual unfolding, and to Judith Aston, who inspired me to take that harmonization a step further and to explore how an aligned body moves. I would like to thank Emily Hilburn Sell and Dave O'Neal of Shambhala Publications for shepherding this book so smoothly through the stages of publication. I would also like to thank Lis Erling Bailly for creating the elegant drawings and symbols.

Many of the structural principles and ideas in this book were first presented in my *Balance of Body, Balance of Mind: A Rolfer's Vision of Buddhist Practice in the West* (Atlanta: Humanics, 1994), and the interested reader who would like to pursue the implications of the posture of meditation further would do well to look there.

The Posture of
Meditation

Introduction

ORDINARILY WE think of meditation as an activity involving our minds, but in truth meditation is initiated by assuming a specific gesture with our bodies. This gesture or posture forms the literal base on which the focused inquiry of meditation ultimately rests and depends. If we build a house with a faulty foundation, we create great difficulties for ourselves when we later take up residence. In the same way, if we do not focus our attention initially on establishing a posture that naturally supports and aids the process of meditation, we create many difficulties for ourselves as we attempt to make progress in our meditative quest.

The word "posture" comes from the Latin *positura,* which means "a position," and *ponere,* "to place." Applied as it customarily is to the structure and appearance of our body, it refers to how we position or place our body in space and to how the different segments of the body relate to one another. In addition, posture or posturing may refer to an attitude or self-image that we self-consciously create, identify with, and project. The determined slouch of an alienated or angry person, the overly developed musculature that attempts to conceal insecurity, the affectation of casual confidence by a lawyer attempting to win over a jury—all of these self-images ultimately depend on holding our bodies in different ways to create a desired effect. By holding our bodies, we create different postures that express different attitudes.

Mostly this kind of posturing or posing carries with it a connotation of unnaturalness. We can tense the muscles in our body and hold ourselves in different postures to manufacture a desired persona or self-image. This is precisely what actors do as they attempt to enter into a role, and consequently theater schools spend a great deal of time focusing on the purely physical aspect of the actor's craft. However, the natural state of the human being, as with any animal, is to be balanced and relaxed. By consciously manipulating our bodies so that we can create and project a specific self-image, we limit our range of expression, restrict the natural movement of energy within our bodies and minds, and forfeit the natural ease of balance and relaxation that is our true birthright.

The French word *poseur* describes this condition quite accurately. It refers to someone who is trying to be something other than what he or she naturally is, an imposter. Contrasted with this unnatural way of being in the body, the posture of meditation aligns our bodies and minds in the most comfortable, guileless way with the greater forces of nature that condition us. In this way we accept ourselves as we are in truth and experience no need to be anything other than what we naturally are already. As we learn to let go of some of our unnatural posturings and posings and enter more comfortably into the posture of meditation, we find that what we naturally are is very wonderful indeed. We experience a comfort and relaxation that reveal ever deeper insights into our true nature.

Just as the gradual, but consistent, evolution of the human

species toward an ever more upright and vertical posture has been accompanied by a parallel growth and expansion in consciousness, so too do the "higher" states of consciousness that can be contacted through the process of meditation themselves depend on the continued refinement of verticality and relaxed balance in the body. This preliminary act of coming to balance as the primary condition on which the inquiry of meditation can proceed is often overlooked, however. Meditation, instead, is mostly presented as a variety of different techniques or activities in which we engage our minds and on which we focus our attention. We may, for example, be instructed to sit and silently repeat a word or phrase or to visualize and merge with the image of a deity. We may be told to sit and pay attention to the passage of breath as it moves in and out of the body or to observe the ever-changing contents of our bodies and minds. We may be asked to sit and attempt to come up with an answer to an insoluble riddle or to imagine a cord of expanding white light in our spines. We may be instructed to sit and listen to the inner sounds of the body or to focus on one particular point in the body to the exclusion of all others. We may sit down and contemplate the meaning of a specific passage from a book we value, or we may simply be instructed to sit and do "nothing at all."

Meditation techniques are extremely varied. The Buddha enumerated approximately forty different techniques, and the *Vigyana Bhairava Tantra* (which Paul Reps translated in *Zen Flesh, Zen Bones*) lists one hundred eight different forms of practice, any of which is capable of taking the practitioner to the highest stages of realization. It is entirely appropriate that there is such a diverse offering of meditation techniques as we all have different temperaments and inclinations that may make one technique a more suitable avenue of exploration for us than others. Many roads can lead to the same place, and ultimately it makes little difference which one we choose as long as it suits our temperament and abilities and allows us to reach our goal. In the end, the best technique is the one we adopt for ourselves.

While the specific techniques of meditation are extremely varied, there exists a denominator common to all of them, and that is the sitting posture itself. It would be very difficult for an observer, even someone who was familiar with the process of meditation, to discern which particular technique a meditator may be practicing. All that the observer can know for sure is that what that person is doing is sitting. Ultimately, the act of sitting itself may become even more important than the technique we are supposedly practicing while sitting. Put another way, techniques themselves may be necessary ways to occupy ourselves as our bodies and minds slowly learn to assume the posture of meditation. Seen this way, the posture of meditation can be viewed as the starting point of the practice as well as its ultimate goal.

Most teachers of meditation do give initial instructions about the importance of posture. These instructions generally take the form of: "Sit with the back straight and the body relaxed. Sit quite still, and breathe comfortably and naturally." The first part of this little volume will be an examination of each part of these instructions and is undertaken in the hopes that it may become much easier for you to put these instructions into practice. As simple as these instructions may be, they also represent one of the most challenging actions that we can attempt to perform. Often if we concentrate on sitting up straight or sitting quite still, we find ourselves becoming rigid, and it becomes very difficult to relax. Or, if we consciously focus on relaxation, we may find that the structure of our bodies slowly begins to collapse. The head begins to hang forward, the front of the body shortens while the back becomes overly elongated, and we lose our verticality. In either of these common positions the natural and comfortable flow of the breath is seriously compromised and impeded. The posture of meditation shows us how to balance and integrate each of these bodily instructions into our sitting practice.

The posture of meditation depends on three primary attributes: alignment, relaxation, and resilience. Each of these attributes is equally important, and each supports the others' manifestation. Appearing together in harmonious relationship to one another, they generate a powerfully catalytic effect on the process of meditation. In this posture the healing energies of the body and mind are naturally activated, and the process of transformation begins spontaneously. Indeed the posture of meditation could be viewed as a *mudra* of transformation, a bodily gesture or attitude through which the process of transformation has no choice but to begin. Whatever personal postural habits of body and mind serve to obscure the truth of our enlightened nature are gradually dissolved through the assumption of this posture, just as the constant unimpeded flow of water gradually dissolves sandstone. We naturally experience this powerfully catalyzing effect as the deepening of our meditation. Body and mind become progressively integrated, and the artificial division between our inner and outer worlds begins to fall away. If any one of these three primary attributes is lacking, the process of meditation may still proceed, but it will do so much more slowly.

The first part of this book will deal with the mechanics of

the posture of meditation as they specifically apply to our formal sitting practice. In the second part of this book we will expand our arena of practice and see how these same principles can be applied to what might be called informal practice, our everyday movements through life. The sections at the end of the chapters are exercises designed to help the reader experience the aspect of the posture of meditation that chapter addresses. A final note: the author's personal form of sitting practice has been strongly influenced by the rich and varied tradition of Buddhism, and indeed references to that tradition will appear from time to time within the text. Even so, the principles underlying the posture of meditation are universal in their application. They apply equally to the meditator who is working with a Theravadin mindfulness practice, a Christian form of contemplation, or a Hindu mystical practice. They apply to all of us who have had the good fortune to recognize that simply to come to sitting can be one of the most potent gestures we are capable of assuming.

Part One

Formal Practice

1

Preliminary Attitudes

IT IS customary to begin a course in meditation by making a formal acknowledgment of the attitudes and forces that can best support the often highly challenging task being undertaken. Within the Buddhist tradition this acknowledgment has taken the form of a declaration that is known as Taking Refuge in the Triple Gem, the three precious jewels or attitudes being the Buddha, or the innate enlightened mind; the Dharma, or the teachings that help us to recontact the enlightened nature of mind; and the Sangha, or the community of fellow practitioners who are treading this path in our company. Whether voiced in the traditional Pali language in which the teachings were first presented or in the contemporary language of the present-day practitioner, the student is asked to recite three times:

> I take refuge in the Buddha.
> I take refuge in the Dharma.
> I take refuge in the Sangha.

With this apparently simple preliminary announcement the practice is begun. The implications of the declaration, however, go far beyond the deceptive simplicity of its form. Contained within this elementary formula are some of the most fundamental of all the teachings that will subsequently be presented. When examined carefully, each of these three components can be seen not only to reveal a correct attitude through which the teachings will reveal themselves, but also to provide hints at the physical postures that will best allow us to embody these attitudes.

The purpose of taking refuge is to seek shelter and protection, to secure the conditions under which we can live safely. While the physical survival of the human body depends on different kinds of physical shelters and conditions, the further nurturance, growth, and maturation of the human being depend on a variety of attitudinal factors that can be cultivated and made manifest through the body and the mind. Just as we must first work to build our homes and secure the foods that protect and nurture our body, so too can we then apply ourselves to creating the conditions that will allow us to experience the fullest potential available to a human being. The preliminary Buddhist act of taking refuge implies that the safety of a human being, seen from the point of view of our personal sanity and well-being, is to be found within the attitudes and forces defined by the Buddha, the Dharma, and the Sangha. Without the protection that is offered by our willingness to open to and embrace these attitudes and forces we stand exposed and in some degree of peril.

Buddha, the first of the three precious attitudes, is not only the appellation given to the historical figure Siddhartha Gautama, a prince from northern India who lived twenty-five hundred years ago and who experienced an extraordinary transformation out of which grew an entire philosophical and psychological system of teaching. It also refers to the enlightened nature of mind and experience that Gautama uncovered in himself and that he knew existed in the form of a seed within every other man and woman as well. While it is normal for every practitioner at some point to develop a profound sense of gratitude and admiration for the pioneering work of the Buddha (or for the primary teacher of whatever lineage of practice they may be exploring), it is the potentially enlightened nature of his or her own mind and experience, not that of the historical Buddha, in which the practitioner is encouraged to take refuge. Indeed Gautama warned against the cult of personality that often develops around a particularly dynamic figure. A reverence for that figure may even interfere with the task facing the individual, the task of becoming a Buddha for oneself. Only through individual perseverance and diligent application of the teachings and techniques can that transformation have a chance of occurring.

Buddha, or the enlightened nature of mind, exists within every one of us. It is not something that we have to manufacture from nothing. It is already there, simply awaiting the conditions that will allow it to appear. Much like the sun that waits patiently to pierce through a dense cloud layer, this aspect of mind waits patiently for our understanding to mature and for the habit patterns that keep its brilliance obscured to drop away. If it did not already exist, it would be hypocritical to expect a student at the very beginning of practice to acknowledge its existence as a refuge and haven of safety. The paradox here is that although the appearance of this aspect of mind is rightly seen as the goal of the practice being undertaken, it is properly viewed as our starting point as well, the point of departure from which the practice is able to unfold.

The justifiable question arises that if this aspect of mind already exists within us, why do we not have freer access to it, why do we not experience it more of the time? Since different states of mind are directly dependent on and produced by specific bodily postures, one answer that presents itself is that we are as yet unable to create and maintain the posture of meditation that naturally supports this condition of mind. When we are able to secure this posture with ease, our conventional state of mind gives way and Buddha, the enlightened nature of mind and experience, suddenly appears. Suzuki Roshi, one of the most respected Buddhist teachers of the twentieth century, has emphasized this correlation between posture and our condition of mind:

> You should not be tilted sideways, backwards, or forwards. You should be sitting straight up as if you were supporting the sky with your head. This is not just form or breathing. It expresses the key point of Buddhism. It is a perfect expression of your Buddha nature. If you want true understanding of Buddhism, you should practice this way. These forms are not a means of obtaining the right state of mind. To take this posture itself is the purpose of our practice. When you have this posture, you have the right state of mind, so there is no need to try to attain some special state.[1]

The defining marks of this posture are a sense of spaciousness, clarity, and calm at the level of mind, and a feeling of subtle, but vibrant, energetic flow at the level of body. So unaccustomed are we to the presence of this quality of experience that it is easier to define by citing the more conventionally familiar aspects of experience that are absent when we successfully assume the posture of meditation. Ordinarily we believe that we are an entity named "I" who lives and resides in our physical body and to whom all experience is ultimately referred. When, however, we open to that place in ourselves to which the term Buddha refers, that aspect of mind for which "I" is an accurate label becomes significantly less substantial. Instead of dominating our sense of self, it recedes to the background of awareness and may even disappear. Whereas formerly we conceived of our body and mind as an object named "I" that moves through space, now we see that at a deeper level of mind from which Buddha emanates we are like space itself through which pass all the components of experience that we can directly perceive through our sensory fields. Our former state of mind and experience was tight, compacted, and claustrophobic. In contrast, the enlightened state of mind and experience is much more expansive, radiant, and spacious.

The key to this transformational shift can be found in the marks of the posture of meditation. A body that is not aligned, relaxed, and resilient creates in itself a great deal of tension and extraneous pain. Any unnecessary tension that exists in the body directly translates itself into tension in the mind. Mentally we feel compressed, compacted, bound in. If, on the other hand, we are able to bring our body into a state of alignment, relaxation, and resilience, then our mind begins to soften and expand as well. If we live in a land that is continually damp and cloudy, we may not believe that anything like the sun, with its warmth, brilliance, and power of penetration, exists at all. Once a break in the clouds has appeared, however, and we have a direct experience of the sun, then we can never more doubt its existence, even when the layer of clouds forms again to conceal it. When we take refuge in Buddha, we are also acknowledging the importance of assuming the posture of meditation. By assuming this posture, we reduce the suffering and pain that are the daily fare of the person whose body is imbalanced, tense, and frozen.

Dharma, the second of the gemlike attitudes that can so valuably assist us, refers to the specific teachings that Gautama developed as a result of the insights that the enlightened nature of his mind revealed to him. The essence of these teachings (as expressed in a series of four short statements called the Four Noble Truths) is that we lock ourselves into a condition of suffering by wanting things to be different from what they are. We may desire things or conditions that do not currently exist; we may be dissatisfied with the ones that do. Any desire keeps us removed from the ability simply to accept ourselves and the conditions in which we find ourselves. The extension to this insight is an obvious one. If we can uproot our constant, frantic tendency to want things to be different, then we can bring an end to the pain and suffering that that tendency constantly creates.

The habit pattern of the body and mind, however, is a formidable foe with which to contend. Constantly clinging to objects or conditions that we desire, constantly reacting with aversion to the ones that we don't, we find it exceedingly difficult simply to accept things as they are. The teachings tell us, however, that while the task may appear justifiably difficult, it is not impossible. An antidote to the pain and suffering that, however subtly, permeate our lives does exist; it is to be found within the refuge of the teachings. The last of the statements that Gautama initially shared was his prescription, presented in the form of a series of techniques and attitudes, for securing that antidote.

Acts of clinging and aversion, no matter how overt or subtle, are expressed through systematic tensing in the musculature of the body. It may seem initially far-fetched to reduce the pain and suffering we experience at the level of mind to what have become virtually involuntary patterns of muscular tensing. Once again, however, we need to remind ourselves that states of mind are dependent on bodily postures. Objects, images, perceptions, thoughts, and attitudes continually come and go in the complex flow of life. Holding on to any of them with the intention that they stay with us forever is dependent on the same kind of muscular tension that we would feel were we to hang on to a long rope that has been secured around the neck of a wild animal. Pushing any of them away with the hope that they will disappear from our lives leaves us feeling equally exhausted and depleted.

Moving constantly back and forth between expressions of pulling and pushing, we bring enormous tension into our body and effectively forfeit our ability to assume the posture of meditation. When our body is tense, it becomes impossible to contact the enlightened nature of mind that the posture of meditation is able, quite naturally, to reveal. It becomes, consequently, even more of a challenge simply to accept ourselves as we are, for when we do we experience a body filled with pain and tension and a mind dominated by the limiting condition "I" with all its attendant likes and dislikes, judgments and passions. Through familiarizing ourselves with the posture of meditation, we can begin to let go of the muscular patterns that lock us into a constant vacillation between the clinging and aversion that cause us so much pain and suffering.

The final force that aids us in our work is the Sangha, the community of others who are undertaking the journey along with us. Ordinarily we do not look to other people as a source of safety and help, viewing them instead with a mixture of fear, mistrust, judgment, and calculation. We may tell ourselves that the welfare of other people is important to us and that we enjoy the warmth and openness of companionship, but often our caring and the degree to which we are willing to be genuinely open and honest are limited. By declaring that our fellow travelers are a source of help and refuge for us, we are forced to reexamine our habitual responses to people. We are also then challenged to change our attitudes toward them when we find our habitual responses limiting our ability to experience others as caring, open, and concerned about our welfare. A leap of faith is required here to initiate this shift in relationship. If we all wait for the other person to demonstrate their goodwill before we respond accordingly, no one ultimately opens, and our hearts remain closed and fearful. If we all simultaneously take the risk to be the first to change the habitual way in which people fearfully respond to one another, then everybody begins to soften, and we all experience the nurturing warmth and benefits that come from a community of people who support one another.

Often we are afraid to share ourselves, our innermost feelings and thoughts, our aspirations and sufferings, out of the fear of ridicule. Indeed, a mind that is locked into fear and jealousy of others (which is a direct function of conceiving of ourselves as an individual "I," separate and distinct from the rest of humanity and the world) will often respond to others with ridicule and some measure of condemnation because of the pain that he or she is feeling. Imagine for a moment, however, a community in which we could give voice to these feelings and thoughts without fear of ridicule and in which we were willing to be open in the most accepting and nonjudgmental way to the feelings and thoughts of the other members. This is the Sangha, or this at least is what the Sangha can aspire and challenge us to.

The teachings can only reveal themselves through a person whose heart is open. The openness of one's heart generates a warmth of feeling that closely correlates to the attributes of the enlightened nature of mind that were previously listed. By opening to our hearts, we exhibit the beginnings of the willingness to accept ourselves as we are. Initially the feelings and sensations that we experience around our heart may appear hardened and dry, laden with heaviness or pain. Gradually, as we continue to open to and accept these feelings, they begin to change. As these feelings and sensations soften and melt, a warmth and spaciousness appear to take their place. It becomes natural to feel caring and concern for the other members of our community, to partake of their joys and successes and to share sympathetically in their unhappinesses and disappointments. As our heart continues to open, a kind of spaciousness begins to permeate our experience. We become "big in heart." As this sense of physical radiation continues to expand, our hardened and fearful outer shells begin to melt away, and it becomes much easier to include others within the enlarged sphere of our immediate experience.

Ordinarily, when we encounter another person, we unconsciously begin to tighten. Rather than opening wider to the encounter, we contract and withdraw our energy in much the same way that a snail retracts its body inside the protective covering of its shell when it senses danger. As we become more sensitive to the tactile changes that are constantly occurring within our body, we can begin to monitor these shifts and come to realize how painful it is to close our hearts and tighten our bodies in the presence of another person, no matter how subtly. If we can begin to view the other person not as a hostile entity to be feared (or at least responded to with caution and care) but as a friend, as a member of our immediate family or Sangha, then we can start experimenting with opening our hearts in the presence of another person.

The opening of the heart is literally dependent on the softening of the musculature around the chest. As Jesus said, "Fortunate are they who have softened the rigidity within, for they can gain access to the universal healing power of Nature."[2] This is a much closer and more literal translation from the original Aramaic language in which Jesus spoke than is the more frequently quoted version, "Blessed are the meek, for they shall inherit the earth." The posture of meditation allows us to begin to soften our rigidities. The more we are able to soften the holding and tightness in our bodies, the easier it is to open our hearts. This cycle feeds on and reinforces itself, for the more our hearts come softly open, the more our bodies shed the tightness and rigidities that make the experience of relaxed and resilient balance so elusive. By closing down our hearts in the presence of our brothers and sisters, we distort our ability to bring our body into a condition of relaxed balance and forfeit the relaxed spaciousness of mind that the posture of meditation offers.

Our attitudes are given literal expression and shape through the tissues and posture of our bodies. By acknowledging the preliminary forces and attitudes that will become our allies in our meditative inquiry, we begin to set in motion the conditions of body and mind that will support our efforts to encourage the posture of meditation to establish itself as our natural, embodied state.

NOTES

1. Shunryu Suzuki, *Zen Mind, Beginner's Mind* (New York and Tokyo: Weatherhill, 1980), p. 26.
2. Neil Douglas-Klotz, *Prayers of the Cosmos* (New York: HarperCollins, 1994), p. 53.

2

Alignment

Sit with the back straight . . .

ANY CHILD who enjoys playing with building blocks understands the principles and importance of alignment. If the blocks are placed one directly on top of the other, the pile remains standing. If the blocks do not bear this vertical relationship to one another, the pile falls over.

These very same principles of alignment determine the degree of balance that is available to a human body. The building blocks of the human body are the major bodily segments: the feet, the lower legs, the upper legs, the pelvis, the abdomen and lower back, the chest and upper back, the shoulders and arms, the neck, and finally, the head. If these segments can be stacked one directly on top of another, that body will be able to stand in a balanced way. A balanced posture requires very little effort to sustain and allows the major muscles of the body to relax. This relatively small expenditure of energy, coupled with the phenomenon of relaxation, produces a distinct feeling tone of softness, ease, and vibratory flow. It also generates a natural condition of alert awareness. This dual condition of comfort in the body and relaxed alertness in the mind is the fruit of balance.

If the major bodily segments are not comfortably stacked one directly on top of the other, the body (unlike the child's blocks) will not topple over, but will have to compensate for its lack of alignment by exerting constant muscular tension to offset the force of gravity. This constant tension generates a feeling tone in the body of hardening, numbness, and pain. It clouds the mind and makes it difficult to remain focused or alert with any kind of ease.

The exact same force provides support for the balanced body and withholds it from the imbalanced body. That force is the gravitational field of the earth. The force of this field always flows through the vertical. Even though the primary function of this most powerful of planetary forces is to draw objects to its source (the center of the earth), it also provides support or buoyancy to any structure that is able to conform its shape to the vertical direction of gravity's flow and influence.

Think for a moment of the giant sequoia trees, the gothic spires of Chartres cathedral, the Eiffel Tower, or the Empire State Building. The tallest trees (nature's oldest living entities) and our tallest buildings are able to reach heights that would not be possible if their structures were not so vertically aligned. The force of gravity supports them by securing their stability. Then think of the Leaning Tower of Pisa. Slowly but surely over the centuries it has continued to lose height, tilting ever more precariously toward its side. In the human body we call this gradual loss of height (and the dulling of mental alertness that all too commonly accompanies it) old age. Is it not possible that there exists a direct correlation between these marks of aging and the fact that a body may never have been fully and successfully able to align itself in such a way as to experience the supporting function of the gravitational field?

If we can find this delicate place in which the uprightness of our body comes into alignment with the vertical flow of gravitational energy, then we experience a natural quality of buoyancy and a feeling of being literally uplifted. If we cannot synchronize the energy field of our body with the vertical flow of gravity, then life can become an exhausting struggle simply to remain erect.

The ability to align the upright structure of the body with the directional flow of gravitational energy is the primary requirement in securing the posture of meditation. Its importance cannot be overemphasized. Our first task, then, is to create a structural situation in which gravity supports our body and meditative efforts. This task corresponds to the initial instructions to "sit with the back straight."

There are three major structural relationships that promote a natural condition of alignment in the posture of meditation. Each relationship builds on the previous one. First of all, the pelvis must be elevated higher than the knees. This allows the pelvis to tip slightly forward so that the weight of the upper body can rest directly above, or even a bit in front of, the sitting bones of the pelvis. The securing of these first two relationships creates a highly stable base of support for the upper body. Situated above such a stable foundation, the upper body can come to a relatively effortless condition of balance as it straightens naturally. The right and left sides of the upper body become approximately symmetrical, while the pelvis, abdomen and lower back, chest and upper back, shoulders, neck, and head stack up one on top of the other just like the child's building blocks.

It may be easier to appreciate just how important these

three structural configurations actually are by examining what happens in the body when these relationships do not exist. Sit for a moment on the floor or in a chair in such a way that your knees are substantially higher than your pelvis. If you let yourself relax in this position, you will notice that your pelvis begins to rock backward over and behind the fulcrum point of your two sitting bones. As your pelvis tips backward in this way, your lower spine begins to shift backward as well. As the lumbar region of your spine moves backward, opposite to its natural curvature, your upper body has no choice but to begin to arc forward in compensation. If you now examine your upper body, you will observe a situation in which the back has become overly elongated while the front of the body has become compressed and shortened. The upper body does not look like a straight, vertical line. It more closely resembles the letter C. There is simply no way for the force of gravity to flow harmoniously through the curvature that has been created by this structural configuration. The result is a body that is not only at odds with gravity, but is also compressing the abdominal viscera and depressing the chest. The compression of the internal abdominal organs does not allow them to function optimally. The compression of the chest significantly inhibits the cycle of breath. The free flow of energy is seriously compromised in such a body. Such a configuration of structure is the somatic equivalent of a knotted garden hose, which seriously impedes the flow of water through it.

You will need to bring a subtle, yet significant and constant, amount of tension into the musculature of the body simply to maintain this position. While the degree of holding may be more prominent and acute in some parts of the body than in others, the overall pattern of holding subtly affects the whole body. The posture of collapse may at first appear to be relaxed, but in actuality it isn't. Within this posture you must constantly brace yourself to offset the pull of gravity. If you were truly to relax and surrender the weight of your body to gravity rather than to brace yourself against it, you might become more compressed and collapsed, crumble even further forward until your head was hanging virtually in your lap, or fall backward. In any case, you cannot relax in this posture and maintain your uprightness.

When we do not experience the force of gravity as a source of support, we must brace and hold ourselves against it. Holding in the body, however, very directly creates holding in the mind. Such holding limits the function of the mind to its most superficial dimensions and will often manifest as an ongoing internal monologue that comments on everything that passes before it and indulges in fantasies about the past and future. The sense of self that accompanies this dimension of the mind will view itself as an entity named "I" separate and distinct from the rest of the world, which it fearfully views as being other than itself and a threat to its existence. Much like a cloud that hides the warming brilliance of the sun, this superficial dimension of the mind effectively conceals the mind's deeper possibilities. It is the superficiality of this most conventional dimension of mind as well as the deeper possibilities that exist beneath this dimension that the process of meditation works to expose and reveal.

All of these difficulties with the posture of collapse began by placing the knees at an elevation higher than the pelvis. Let's see what begins to happen when this relative positioning is reversed. You may choose once again to sit cross-legged on the floor or in a chair. This time, however, place enough

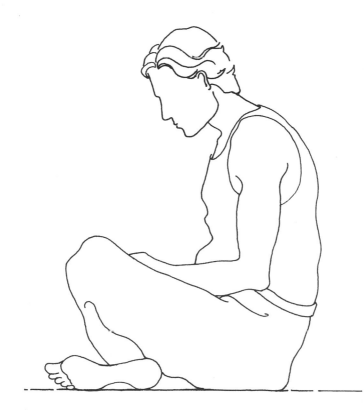

If the knees are higher than the sitting bones, the pelvis and lumbar spine must shift backward, and the upper torso assumes a posture of collapse. Like a knotted garden hose that obstructs the passage of water flowing through it, a collapsed body is unable to allow the life force to move freely through its length. Obstruction to the free and unimpeded passage of the life force causes the energy of the body and mind to alternate between periods of sluggishness and agitation.

firm, supporting cushions underneath your pelvis to ensure that your pelvis is higher than your knees. In this position the top of your pelvis naturally comes a bit forward. Your cushions will now contact the very bottom of your sitting bones, or you may find that your point of contact is even a bit in front of the bottom of your sitting bones.

As your pelvis tips forward, it brings your lumbar spine forward with it. This is the natural position for the lumbar spine to assume. The thoracic portion of your spine is then able to assume its natural slight curvature backward. The cervical portion of your spine comes slightly forward, and the head is able to balance quite effortlessly on top of it all. When teachers of meditation speak of sitting with the spine straight, they don't mean that these natural curves should be flattened. These slight curves occur at the approximate points where several of the major energy centers or chakras have been traditionally cited as being positioned. When these curves are comfortably situated, the body can begin to relax, and through this relaxation these centers can naturally begin to open and blossom.

When the sacral, lumbar, thoracic, and cervical regions of the spine are able to assume the slight curvature natural to them, the upper body becomes vertical and upright. The right and left sides of the body appear to hang symmetrically off of the vertical axis that has been established in the very center of the torso. The length of the front of the body appropriately matches the length of the back of the body. Maximum space is created in the abdomen for the internal abdominal organs to settle comfortably. Restrictions to the immediate structures involved in the action of breathing are minimized as well.

Just as the tallest trees and skyscrapers appear to stand

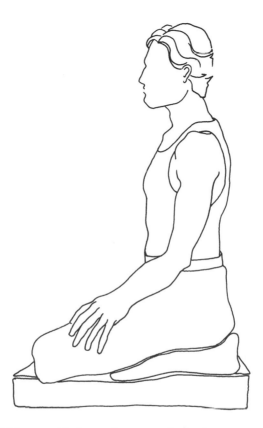

By establishing a stable base of support, the body naturally comes into alignment with the directional flow of gravity. Once alignment has been established, the body can begin to become relaxed and resilient. The deeply purifying process of meditation has no choice but to begin.

effortlessly, so too can the sitting meditator experience a place of calm and stability through bringing the body into vertical alignment in this way. Because the verticality of structures is supported by the force of gravity, over time the meditator will come to realize how extraordinarily comfortable this posture feels. It is important to stress that the posture of meditation is not a contrived or contorted positioning of the body whose purpose is to generate unusual insights or states of consciousness. On the contrary, once we are comfortably able to find and assume this posture and begin to experience the buoyant support of gravity, a distinct feeling tone of naturalness and authenticity begins to appear. We begin to realize that the posture of meditation reveals not some extraordinary condition of the body and mind, but rather the natural state that is available to us as our birthright. Through aligning our body with the vertical flow of the force of gravity, we begin quite literally to experience the support of the larger universe of which we are but a small part.

Alignment that conforms to the directional flow of gravity has a distinct feeling tone of rightness to it. This feeling tone, or lack of it, becomes our primary guide as we attempt to find this place of alignment and bring it into our sitting posture. If we sit in front of a mirror and consciously manipulate the various parts of our body to conform to the vertical, we may unwittingly bring more tension into our sitting posture. This is like attempting to superimpose alignment onto the structure of the body from the outside in. If, however, we simply generate the three primary gestures of alignment (the pelvis higher than the knees; the very bottom, or even a place just in front of the very bottom, of the sitting bones contacting the cushion; the upper torso balancing itself as effortlessly as possible over the stable base of support created by the first two gestures) and then allow the body to make whatever adjustments in posture spontaneously occur, the feeling tone of alignment gradually and inevitably begins to emerge. Paying more attention to the feeling tone of alignment rather than to its spatial coordinates allows us to align ourselves with gravity from the inside out.

Because every body is unique, there can be no specific rules as to how much higher the pelvis should be than the knees. You will need to experiment with different thicknesses of supporting cushions (or heights of kneeling benches) until you find the combination that is appropriate for your body. Over time, as the posture of your meditation continues to refine itself, this combination may have to be adjusted. Stay sensitive to the feeling tones of balance. They will provide you with continuous information that will allow you to determine whether or not your body is continuing to move in the direction of alignment.

The three primary gestures of alignment apply equally whether you are sitting on a kneeling bench, in a chair, or cross-legged on the floor. If the tradition of practice to which you are drawn so allows, experiment with different ways of sitting. To sit in the traditional cross-legged posture you will want a broad supporting foam pad to ease the strain you might otherwise feel in your knees and ankles in addition to the individual cushions to raise the height of your pelvis. How you cross your legs depends largely on the degree of flexibility at your ankle, knee, and hip joints as well as on the length of your upper and lower legs. If you have a great deal of natural flexibility, the traditional full lotus posture, in which not only do your legs cross each other but your feet come to rest on the top of the opposite thigh, may be very comfortable and stable. If this is not comfortable (and for a majority of people it will not be), there is no need to force your legs into this position. You may choose instead to cross one leg loosely over the other or sit with one leg in front of the other. The ability to sit in full lotus does not in itself confer any status of greater attainment. It is more a function of body mechanics than anything else. Again, pay most attention to the feeling tones in your body. Find the cross-legged position that is the most comfortable for you to assume. The position that you find will be different from the position your neighbor finds.

Almost inevitably you will discover that it is much easier to cross one leg over the other, rather than the other way around. For example, you may be quite comfortable with your right leg crossed loosely over your left, but find that reversing the position and crossing your left over your right is significantly less comfortable and may even distort the alignment of your upper body. If this is the case, it is quite important that you change the placement of your legs (right over left, left over right) from one sitting to the next. In the beginning spend much less time in the less comfortable position, but over time keep working with both until your body has adjusted itself and released some of its holding and you can sit equally comfortably with your legs crossed either way. A time may even come when the formerly uncomfortable positioning of the legs can actually become more stable than the initial comfortable placement. In this way the sitting posture helps us to release the structural imbalances that exist in the body. As the body becomes more naturally balanced, it becomes much easier to maintain the posture of meditation not only in the formal sitting posture, but as we move through life as well.

The placement of the hands in the formal posture of meditation is best determined not by any specific rule, but by the relationship between the lengths of the arms and the torso. Again this will be different for everyone. Cupping one hand loosely in the other and resting them both on the lap may be quite comfortable for someone whose arms are quite long relative to the length of his or her torso, but not nearly so comfortable for someone with a long torso and relatively short arms. Some people will find placing the hands lightly on the knees much more comfortable than will other people. Again, the key is comfort. Experiment with different placements until you find the positioning that is the most comfortable for your body. In the upright human form arms are designed to hang, completely surrendered to the pull of gravity. Any placement of the arms within the formal posture of meditation that inhibits this surrender will cause holding or tightening through the shoulder girdle and consequent interference with the free flow of breath and energy through the body.

Establishing alignment through synchronizing the structure of the upright torso with the directional flow of the force of gravity is the first key in establishing the posture of meditation. It is the foundation on which the next two keys—relaxation and resilience—ultimately rest and depend. If we do not first bring our awareness to establishing alignment in our sitting posture, our ability to relax and be resilient in that posture will be significantly compromised.

Shortly before the Buddha experienced his enlightenment, he met a grass-cutter who gave him a bushel of straw with which to make his meditation seat more comfortable. It is reported that the Buddha graciously accepted this gift, arranged his seat, and renewed his efforts. A bushel of straw on which to sit may not seem like much to us, accustomed as we are to the ready availability of high density foams or natural fiber cushionings. Twenty-five hundred years ago, however, a bushel of straw quite probably represented a significant gift. It is tempting to imagine that the Buddha was able to craft the straw into a supporting cushion that not only provided greater comfort but, even more important, also raised his pelvis to a higher elevation than his knees, allowing his upper body to align itself much more comfortably with the directional flow of gravity. It was not long after receiving this gift that the Buddha's long search and inquiry experienced a final acceleration that would culminate in his full enlightenment.

To bring alignment into our sitting posture we need to organize the mass of the upper body as economically as possible around an imaginary vertical axis that runs through the center of our torso. This vertical axis is imaginary in that it does not correspond to any specific anatomical structure; it does, however, correspond precisely to the directional flow of the force of gravity. By efficiently organizing our body around this axis we create a situation in which gravity is able to reinforce the uprightness of our posture. Any major structural deviations, either to the right or the left of this axis, or in front of or behind it, will present gravity with a mass on which it must exert its pull and influence. We will then have to brace ourselves against this pull and compromise the degree of relaxation and resilience that alignment otherwise makes possible. The purpose of creating alignment is to create a situation in which gravity can work for us rather than against us. As we begin to experience gravity as a source of support, we will come to realize that this support is not just experienced as a mechanical function. A profound process of healing, at the levels of both the body and the mind, spontaneously begins to occur for the person who is able to synchronize the alignment of the body with the directional flow of gravity.

Begin by sitting in your customary meditation posture. You may be sitting cross-legged on the floor, on a kneeling bench, or in a chair. If you choose to sit on a chair, sit well to the front and do not lean against the back of the chair. Examine the sensations in your body generated by your posture. How comfortable and supported do you feel in your posture? Are there parts of the body that feel as though they have to tense and brace themselves, to hold on to maintain the uprightness of your posture and to prevent your falling over? See if you can locate and identify these places if they do, in fact, exist. Over time we become accustomed to the holding and tension in our body. We experience them as normal. Examine some of these places calmly and slowly. See if you can detect the holding that can be felt to exist there. Can you simply let go of the holding that you discover by relaxing the tension in the muscle group that is creating it? What happens to your posture if you are able to do this?

Now turn your attention to the relationship between the height of your pelvis and the height of your knees. Begin to add as many supporting cushions as necessary to bring your pelvis to a higher elevation than your knees. Closely watch how the addition of supporting cushions affects the angle of your pelvis, the point of contact between your sitting bones and your seat, and the position of your lumbar spine. Invariably you will find that your pelvis tilts forward, the lumbar spine also moves forward, and the point of contact between your sitting bones and your seat shifts forward as well.

Keep experimenting with different thicknesses or numbers of supporting cushions. Too thin or two low a supporting cushion will not allow the pelvis, lumbar spine, and point of contact of the sitting bones to shift forward sufficiently to function as a stable base of support for the upper body. Too high a supporting cushion will cause the pelvis to shift too far forward and create a condition of swayback in the lumbar spine. Too high a pelvis is just as capable of compromising the base of support on which your alignment depends as is too low a pelvis. Feel what happens in your body when you sit on no supporting cushions. Feel what happens in your body when you sit on too many supporting cushions. Slowly keep experimenting, adding or removing cushions as necessary, until you find a place between these two extremes that begins to feel comfortable and over which your torso begins to experience a greater ease of balance.

Once you have created a stable base of support, you can turn your attention to your torso. Visualize the major bodily segments of your torso—the abdomen and lower back, the chest and upper back, the shoulders and arms, the neck, and the head—as a grouping of interdependent building blocks. Any adjustment to the positioning of any one of these units will inevitably affect the stability and placement of all the others. Visualize the segments of your upper body stacked comfort-

ably and efficiently one on top of the other, and then slowly
allow your body to reposition itself so as to approximate your
visualization. Let the feelings and sensations of your body initiate and guide this subtle readjustment. Alignment has a distinct feeling tone of rightness and buoyancy to it. Release any
tensions that may enter into the readjustment of your posture.
The alignment that you seek is a completely natural and comfortable condition. It is not an artificial and rigid condition
like the standing military posture.

Now begin to sway slightly. Move the upper body forward
and back and from one side to the other. Let this swaying
movement be natural, relaxed, and easy. The whole upper
body can move together as an integrated unit composed of
interdependent parts. Let the legs remain relatively immobile
during this exercise, and initiate the movement in the pelvis.
The major joint, then, out of which the movement will be
initiated will be the place where the upper legs (specifically,
the greater trochanters of the femurs) come into contact with
the socket joints of the pelvis. Move randomly, perhaps
bringing circular or figure-eight motions into your movement. In the beginning let the movements be quite noticeable and imagine that the upper body is swaying around an
imaginary vertical axis like streamers around a maypole.
Gradually decrease the range of motion, making the movements around the vertical axis smaller and subtler. Keep making the movements smaller and smaller until it feels as though
they have completely stopped.

Now slowly begin to move your upper body quite far to the
left. Let the fulcrum of this movement be your anatomical

waistline. As your upper body moves to the left, you may feel your pelvis shift slightly to the right as a counterbalance. If your hands are resting with the palms facing down on your knees, you will feel your right hand slide toward your body and your left hand slide away from your body as you do this. Move as far as possible without straining. Let your shoulders, arms, neck, and head hang comfortably in this position.

When you have moved your upper body as far to the left as possible, slowly begin to reverse the direction of your movement. The upper body will come back to center and, without stopping, continue moving to the right. The pelvis will shift back to center and move slightly to the left. Your right hand will slide slightly forward on your knee as your left hand slides back. Let your movements be as fluid as possible. Breathe easily and comfortably throughout the movement.

Keep moving slowly back and forth, exploring the limits of your body's range of motion to the right and to the left. Pay special attention to the feelings and sensations that this movement generates in the body. You may be able to detect an intensification of sensations as the upper torso moves as far as possible to the right or to the left. As you move back to center, this intensification will be experienced to lessen. Just before you begin to move past center to the other side you may be able to detect a significant lightening quality to the sensations.

Now begin to decrease the range of your movements to the left and to the right, paying ever more attention to the subtle lightening of sensations that occurs in the center of this movement. Let the movements become smaller and smaller until they gradually come to a stop around this centermost point. This point is your vertical axis through which the force of gravity naturally flows, and it possesses a distinct, and quite recognizable, feeling tone.

Now begin a slow, undulating, rocking movement of the spine backward and forward. Initiate this movement with the pelvis. Begin by very slowly rocking your pelvis backward so that you contact your cushion far behind the midpoint of your sitting bones. As you do this, start allowing the rest of your spine to respond naturally and accordingly. The lumbar and lower thoracic portions of your spine will shift backward in response. The upper thoracic portion of your spine, your neck, and finally your head will begin to drop forward. Explore the sensations, as well as the quality of mind, that this hyperflexed posture of collapse creates in your body. After a few seconds begin to reverse the movement. Initiate this reversal of position once again with your pelvis. As you begin slowly and sensitively to rock your pelvis as far forward as possible, your spine will begin to uncoil and come out of its collapsed position. The lumbars will move forward, the front of the chest and the neck will lengthen and expand, and the head will tilt backward as the eyes look up toward the place where the wall joins the ceiling. Be very careful not to strain. Take a few comfortable breaths in this hyperextended position, and then slowly begin reversing it again by initiating a movement backward in your pelvis.

Continue this slow, undulating movement forward and backward several times. Let the movement be as fluid, sinuous, and coordinated as possible. Gradually begin to decrease the range of movement backward and forward. The body will become less collapsed in its forward flexed position and less extended in its backward position. As you continue to make your movements smaller and smaller, make sure that you maintain the fluidity and coordination inherent in this undulating motion. Gradually you will come to a place where the forward and backward movement effectively ceases. Pay special attention to the feeling tone in your body as you come to this place as once again you have brought your body into a much closer alignment with the imaginary vertical axis through which the force of gravity naturally flows.

The posture of meditation is not a static position that we search to discover and then maintain. It is, rather, a deeply organic process that will naturally evolve and shift over time as your sense of balance becomes increasingly refined. As you work to bring the condition of alignment into your sitting posture, keep monitoring the ever-changing sensations of your body. They will provide the data that will help you to keep moving in the direction of ever greater alignment. Keep feeling your body as it is. From moment to moment this feeling may change. Spontaneous adjustments in posture may begin to occur. These adjustments may appear in the form of smooth or even jerky movement. Allow these adjustments. Yield to them. This is the body's way of becoming ever more balanced as we continue to align ourselves with the force of gravity.

3

Relaxation

. . . and the body relaxed.

RELAXATION IS a function of the body's ability to surrender its weight to the pull of gravity. If we are constantly bracing ourselves against the force of gravity, we cannot truly relax. This is why alignment is so crucial as the first step in establishing the posture of meditation. The upright structure of an aligned body, much like a tall tree or skyscraper, is both supported and stabilized by the force of gravity. Consequently there is no need for it to brace itself against anything. It can completely surrender its weight to the pull of gravity, and still it remains standing.

If the body is not so vertically aligned, we must instead rely on muscular tension to support us. The primary purpose of this muscular tension is to counteract the downward pull of gravity. Visualize for a moment a situation in which the head is angled forward of the ideal midline of the body. The muscles of the back of the neck and upper back must constantly contract to offset the negative influence of gravity. If we were to relax these muscles, the head and neck would fall even further forward and down, and ultimately the body might topple to the ground. If, however, the head sits directly on top of an aligned body like the topmost building block in a child's tower, the muscles of the back of the neck and upper back can relax. They do not have to exert any unnecessary muscular tension to keep the head balanced on top of the rest of the body. Within this condition of relaxation the head (and the rest of the aligned body as well) can surrender its weight to the pull of gravity without forfeiting its uprightness.

By aligning our body with the directional flow of the gravitational field, we effectively transform the effect of gravity from a force against which we must constantly struggle and brace ourselves into a force that can provide both support and stabilization, a sea in which we can float and feel buoyed up. Gravity, then, is simply a neutral force. Depending on the structure on which it interacts, however, it may be experienced positively or negatively.

Relaxation without alignment can only be partial at best. Alignment without relaxation creates a condition of great rigidity much like the soldier at boot camp standing tensely at attention. The standing military posture seeks to create good soldiers. By bringing a great deal of tension into his body, the soldier is effectively able to lessen the awareness of his sensations and feelings. Through limiting his awareness and impulses, he becomes much more amenable to following orders and doing the bidding of his superior officers.

The posture of meditation, however, seeks to create the conditions in which meditative inquiry can come to fruition. While different traditions of spiritual practice will express the goal of meditation through different metaphors, all forms of practice are designed to help the student come to a deeper understanding of the nature of reality. The ultimate nature may be expressed as an awareness of Christ's love, the discov-

ery of one's natural state, the attainment of the enlightened
condition, or the simple ability to see things as they actually
are. The primary tool that helps us in any of these undertak-
ings is a sharply honed awareness that can be directed to examine objects of experience both inside and outside our
bodies. Maintaining chronic tension in the body, however, is
the most effective way in which we can block out awareness
of whole levels of experience. Then, no matter how penetrating our awareness may be, there is little for it to examine.
By locking our body into patterns of tension and rigidity, we
become numb to our sensations and feelings. We restrict the
full flow and natural expression of our breath. We fail to hear
all the sounds that are happening around and inside us; the
visual field can rapidly lose its sense of luminosity, color, and
three-dimensionality. As we continue to lose awareness of
these most primary manifestations of reality, our internal
monologue builds in strength and intensity. As we listen to
the often skewed and highly subjective pronouncements of
this monologue, we even further remove ourselves from an
objective awareness of the nature of reality.

By relaxing through surrendering the weight of the body
to the pull of gravity, we allow unnecessary tension in the
body literally to fall away. As the musculature of the body
continues to relax, we become much more aware of our sensations and feelings. Formerly the tension in the musculature
created a kind of armoring that prevented us from fully feeling the tactile sensations in our bodies. As we relax this tension, we are often flooded by the awareness of these
sensations, and we become able to experience the body as it
is. The relaxation of tension also enables us to hear and see
with greater clarity, and the internal monologue of the mind
naturally begins to subside. As we learn to experience the

components of reality (our sensations, sights, sounds, tastes, smells, and thoughts) with greater ease and precision, we naturally begin penetrating to an awareness of ever deeper levels of that reality.

Just as the importance of posture is often overlooked in spiritual practice, so too is the ability to accept and experience the body as it is. In many spiritual traditions the body is presented as an impediment to attainment. Attachment to, and identification with, the body are seen as one of the major obstacles to experiencing the goals of the practice. One of the unfortunate consequences of this understanding, however, has been to bring a great deal of tension and holding into the body as an unconscious strategy to break one's attachment to the body by blocking out awareness of it. The creation of tension and holding, however, can only serve to fuel our identification with the superficial dimension of the mind that the practice is ostensibly designed to dissolve.

On every part of the body down to the smallest cell tactile sensations can be felt to exist. Even though these sensations are almost unimaginably small in size and are appearing and dissolving with astonishing rapidity, their presence can be distinctly felt. If you hold out your hand with the palm up, allow it to relax, and focus your awareness there, you will begin to feel a mass of tingling sensations in the hand as though a current of minute vibrations is flowing through the hand. These sensations exist on every part of the body all the time, but ordinarily we are very rarely aware of them. The holding and tension in the musculature of the body effectively blocks out our awareness of this experiential dimension of our bodies. This same holding and tension then fuels the activity of the superficial level of our minds. A condition of profound relaxation can begin quite dramatically to reverse this polarity. As we become more aware of the body as a unified field of tactile sensations, the activity of our inner monologue simultaneously begins to diminish.

By creating a condition of alignment, we can begin to relax our bodies and minds. As the feeling of relaxation expands and tension and holding are felt to fall away, we are able to penetrate to deeper and deeper levels of awareness. As we come face to face with the deepest realities of our bodies and minds, we are then challenged to let go of our conceptions or notions of identity and align our sense of self instead with the experience that our condition of alignment and relaxation have revealed. Paradoxically, the awakening of the awareness of body as a unified field of constantly changing, shimmering sensations becomes the doorway through which our conventional understanding of the body as a physical object separate and distinct from the rest of reality, an object that we then attach ourselves to and identify ourselves with, is revealed to be incorrect.

Furthermore, the current of sensations that can be felt to flow through the body rapidly becomes a powerful source capable of dissolving physical blockages that may exist in the body and of purifying the mind of its residual patterns of limiting thoughts. The twentieth-century Burmese meditation teacher U Ba Khin spoke of this force as *nibbana dhatu,* a force capable of cleansing the body and mind of blockage and impurity and revealing the awareness of the enlightened state in its place. Through entering into a profound process of relaxation the meditator is able to kindle an awareness of the whole body as a field of tactile sensations. These sensations, then, can be experienced to form a current or force. It is as though the physical body becomes a conduit or a position in space through which the current of sensations, the life force of the body, flows. It is not technically accurate to say that this force flows through the body because it also *is* the body. A body that can align itself with gravity and then relax through surrendering its weight to the pull of gravity activates an awareness of its tactile, sensational presence. This presence, then, becomes a force that itself can purify the body and mind and reveal the meditative awarenesses that are the goal of the practice.

If the conditions of alignment and relaxation are not brought into the posture of meditation, this process of purification will still occur, but it will do so very much more slowly. A sandstone boulder that falls into a river will gradually be dissolved by the action of the water that passes over and around it. Imagine, however, that there is a logjam just downstream from where the boulder has settled. The water will be moving very slowly in this area of the river. The slower the current moves, however, the softer will be the abrasive action of the water on the sandstone boulder. If the logjam can be cleared and the current of the river increased, the abrasive action of the water on the sandstone boulder will increase dramatically, and the boulder will dissolve much more quickly. In much the same way the posture of meditation is able to generate a pronounced, catalytic effect on the process of meditation. The key to this acceleration is relaxation. Alignment is only important in so far as it allows us to surrender the weight of the body to the pull of gravity and experience the feeling of relaxation.

To relax in this way is to reestablish your connection with the earth. Through real relaxation the energy field of the body merges compatibly and harmoniously into the greater gravitational energy field of the earth. Relaxation, then, is synonymous with grounding. True grounding occurs not just through feeling the connection between the feet and the ground, but rather through feeling the whole body as a unified field of sensation surrendering its weight to the gravitational pull underneath its feet.

Many years ago a young meditation student attended a weekend retreat at a recently opened Tibetan dharma center. The student arrived not only with an assortment of pillows on which to sit, but with pencils and paper with which to write down what he assumed would be highly complex and esoteric meditation instructions. Imagine his profound surprise when, after assuming a sitting posture, the whole of the instructions to follow consisted of one word alone: *relax*. That one word was repeated again and again over the entire weekend, and no other instructions were given.

It may be easier to contact the experience of surrendering the weight of your body to the pull of gravity if you begin by lying down on your back. You may lie on the floor, on a mat or bed, or on the ground. Begin by simply resting. Take at least a minute to let your body settle down onto the surface that supports it, and allow your breath to breathe you in whatever pattern it naturally assumes. Do not forcibly try to change anything: your pattern of breath, your level of relaxation, the sensations you may be experiencing. If these change on their own, simply allow that change to occur, but do not feel that you need to change anything about your experience. Relaxation occurs through allowance, a literal giving in to forces that are much more powerful than you. Forcing relaxation to occur is a contradiction in terms.

Gently move your attention to your right foot, and simply allow whatever tension or holding you find in your right foot to let go and relax. Feel how your right foot can surrender itself to gravity. Feel what happens as you allow this surrender to occur. Take however much time you need. As you let go of residual tension through surrendering a part of the body to gravity, you will experience an immediate shift in the nature of the tactile sensations in that part of the body. Once that shift has occurred, you can move your awareness to a different part.

Move your attention in turn to your right lower leg, your right upper leg, your left foot, your left lower leg, your left upper leg. Feel how each part of the body that you are focusing on can be experienced to let go and release subtle tension as you surrender that part to the omnipresent pull of gravity. Observe the difference in the tactile sensations of each part of the lower body after you have allowed this surrender to occur.

Continue moving your awareness up the body. Feel the entire basin of the pelvis soften and let go, the abdomen and lower back, the chest and upper back. Move your attention to the right shoulder, the right upper arm, the right lower arm, the right hand. Once you have experienced a distinct shift in sensations, turn your attention to your left shoulder, upper and lower arm, and hand. Feel the throat and the neck surrender to gravity. Feel each part of the body as though it were an object that a child was holding in her hand and simply released. Feel the face and the head let go in the same way.

Acknowledge how different the body feels in this relaxed state. The breath may have shifted on its own. The activity of the mind may also have slowed down significantly. Move your awareness briefly through your body a second time. Can you allow the individual body parts to release even further? In a condition of complete surrender the mind may stop completely. Notice what has happened in the body when the thought process resumes again. Inevitably the resumption of involuntary thought is accompanied by the reappearance of tension and resistance to gravity in some part of the body as well.

In this very relaxed state you will be much more aware of the whole body as a unified field of tactile sensations. These sensations may be very noticeable or extremely subtle, a scarcely detectable shimmer. As you experience the whole body as a surrendered unit, notice how these sensations form a kind of active current or force that appears to pass through you from top to bottom and back again. Visualize the physical body as a completely relaxed, hollow bamboo tube through which the energy of your life force can freely and organically move and circulate in whatever pattern is appropriate to it at that moment. Notice how this life force can be felt to ebb and flow, how it builds one moment and subsides the next in a random pattern of manifestation that is deeply organic and unpredictable. Feel how the perimeter of the channel in which this current flows is not just limited to the surface of your physical body, but that it can actually be felt to radiate out from the physical body. Keep surrendering the weight of the body to gravity, accepting whatever states of awareness and consciousness naturally occur as you allow this process to continue.

After spending some time lying down, familiarizing yourself with the feeling and process of relaxation, you may want to come up to sitting. Assume your formal posture of meditation, and begin by bringing a condition of alignment into your posture through exploring the exercises at the end of the previous chapter. Once you have experienced the maximum amount of alignment available to you at this time, turn your attention back to the process of relaxation. The alignment of your body will allow you to surrender your weight to the pull of gravity quite freely without toppling over, so begin to relax and let go as fully as possible.

You may wish to begin by taking a number of deep breaths. On your last exhalation turn your attention back to the tactile sensations in your body, allowing your breath to assume whatever pattern is natural to it. You may wish once again to move your attention part by part through the entire body, contacting the feelings and sensations in that part of the body and then allowing the taste and experience of relaxation to enter into that part of the body as you surrender its weight to the pull of gravity. Begin by bringing your attention to the top of the head, your scalp, and forehead. Feel whatever tension or residual holding you may find there begin to melt away, yielding to the ever present pull of gravity. Relax the eyes. You may wish to close them lightly. If the eyes want to stay open, observe the sensations in and around your eyes quite carefully, making sure that you are not inadvertently creating tension by focusing too precisely on a specific object or distance. Slowly bring the feeling of relaxation to your cheeks and ears, your nose, your jaw, your mouth and your chin. As you do this, the mouth may naturally want to hang slightly open. Bring your awareness to the area around your tongue, and feel that this area too can yield to the subtle pull of gravity. Feel the entire head aligned on top of the body and relaxed.

It may be helpful to remember that the head weighs approximately ten pounds. If it is not balanced on top of the supporting torso, the muscles in the neck and upper back will have to contract to keep the head in that position. Many meditators have a tendency to let the head drop forward and to look slightly down at the floor. This tendency also creates tension in the neck and the shoulders. When the head is aligned and relaxed, the eyes look straight ahead.

Ordinarily the area of the head may be completely occupied by the presence of involuntary thought. In a deeply relaxed and balanced condition, however, the head can experience a full range of tactile sensations filling and occupying its space. Sensation and involuntary thought cannot occupy the same space simultaneously. Where do the thoughts go when the head is able to experience itself as a mass of sensations? Where do the sensations go when you become distracted by thought? Explore the role that relaxation plays in the creation of these two different states.

Continue moving your attention through each and every part of the body. Feel how you can release tension in the throat and the back and sides of the neck by gently surrendering the weight in this part of your body to gravity. If you discover any unexpected tension, do not try to force it away. Simply spend a bit longer in that part of the body, patiently continuing to allow the tension in that part to drop away. Move your awareness to your shoulders, your arms, your hands, your chest and upper back, your belly and lower back, your pelvis, your legs, and your feet. You may even be able to feel the dropping away of tension like water in a shower that runs down your body. As you let go of tension in any one part of the body, the experience of relaxation in other parts of your body may be affected as well. As your body becomes increasingly relaxed, you may experience a refinement to your alignment as well. Allow these shifts to continue to occur. In a deeply relaxed state the sensations in the entire body can be felt to ebb and flow. As your alignment subtly shifts through this deep relaxation, watch to make sure that you have not inadvertently brought any additional tension anywhere into the body. As you continue to surrender your weight to the pull of gravity, keep playing with your balance. In the posture of meditation you may ultimately be able to find a place of balance that requires no unnecessary effort at all to maintain.

Keep moving your awareness through your body, continuing to relax even more. Once you have kindled a relaxed awareness of the entire body, you may choose to focus on only a few places to maintain the ongoing process of relaxation. A convenient formula that can remind you of this says simply: drop your shoulders, drop your belly, drop your mind, open your heart.

Koans are apparently insoluble riddles that students in the Rinzai school of Japanese Buddhism are, nonetheless, required to solve as part of their meditation practice. "What is the sound of one hand clapping?" one student may typically be asked. He or she is then sent off to ponder the koan during long hours of sitting meditation in hopes of arriving at an answer to a question that is essentially unanswerable.

On the face of it, the task of resolving the dilemma posed by the koan appears impossible. One hand alone can't clap, and it certainly wouldn't be able to make any sound if it could. We are clearly not dealing within the realm of the logical world here. The purpose of the koan, however, is to free us from the restrictions that that realm ordinarily imposes, to force us to look at things in a radically different way. Faced with an apparently impossible situation, our customary mental conditioning may have no recourse but to shut itself down, revealing in its place a wonderfully refreshing dimension of experience that is extremely difficult to access under normal conditions. In the words of Hakuin, one of the great koan masters, "If you take up one koan and investigate it unceasingly, your mind will die."

The orientation of traditional koan practice is decidedly mental, and the struggle to resolve the koan takes place entirely within the mind of the student. However, just as we have conventional patterns of the mind that serve to obscure some of the deeper, more wholesome dimensions of experience, so too do we have conventional ways of being in the body that limit and restrict us to a diminished condition of vitality and ease. And just as the mind can be presented, for the purposes of awakening, with puzzles or riddles that initially appear impossible to resolve, so too can the body be presented with tasks that at first appear to be contradictory and impossible to perform.

The posture of meditation itself may appear as a kind of somatic koan. Alignment and relaxation would initially seem to be contradictory impulses. We can easily imagine a soldier standing at attention, erect and straight. We can also easily imagine someone lying on the beach, completely relaxed. The synthesizing of these two impulses into one compatible gesture, however, is much more difficult to visualize, and yet this is what the posture of meditation challenges us to accomplish. The effect of combining alignment with relaxation goes far beyond a mere functional improvement of the body. Just as with the traditional koan, a wonderfully wholesome dimension of experience that is ordinarily elusive and difficult to access may spontaneously present itself. The koan may be simply stated:

> In a sitting or standing position surrender the entire weight of the body to gravity, and yet remain as tall as you possibly can be.

The exploration of this koan goes far beyond the simple securing of a stable posture. Unlike the inanimate materials that are used in the construction of tall buildings, the tissues and cells of the human body are animated by a life force that adds an extraordinarily dynamic element completely lacking in the steel girders that form the backbone of a modern skyscraper. While this inner force is always present, its fullest expression remains dormant or contained in most humans. One of the simplest explanations for this restriction is that the holding and muscular tensing that are necessary to keep an imbalanced body standing erect effectively serve to contain that force and render it inactive. However, if a human body is able to come to balance not by exerting unnecessary muscular effort, but by establishing a predominantly vertical structure, then that body can begin to liberate this force. As a balanced body continues to surrender its weight to gravity, this force becomes activated, and the body may gradually and quite spontaneously begin to feel as if it is being gently elongated and stretched upward and outward. This elongation and stretching are the natural manifestation of this life force. In the life cycle of plants this force is responsible for drawing the body of the plant upward in the direction of the sky. In human beings this force can be felt as a source of extension or radiation. When, through a gesture of profound relaxation, this force is activated, it may initially cause chills in the body, or the body may tremble or quiver. Sometimes it may almost feel as if you are being drawn up by some mysterious force analogous to the force of gravity, yet opposite to it in its direction of pull and influence. When mystics speak of feeling uplifted or drawn closer to God, it is the activation of this inner bodily force that is responsible. To arrive at this experience is to resolve the apparent contradiction posed by the koan and to begin to appreciate the depth of wisdom embodied in the posture of meditation.

4

Resilience

Sit quite still, and breathe comfortably and naturally.

WHEN WE sit down in meditation, we are instructed to sit very still like an unmoving mountain or a carved statue of Buddha, to let go of extraneous motions, gestures, or nervous movement habits. Stillness, however, is antithetical to life. The common denominator to all life forms is the presence of motion. Everything is moving. Everything is pulsing. This is as true of individual cells as it is of large vertebrate mammals. True stillness and immobility only enter into our bodies when we die. The posture of meditation is able to reconcile this apparent contradiction between stillness and motion through adding the element of resilience to the preliminary conditions of alignment and relaxation.

It is important to recognize that, when applied as a value to the process of meditation, stillness refers to the gradual softening and quieting of the body and mind. It does not imply rigidity or immobility. The stillness of meditation, rightly understood and experienced, promotes the quality of quiescence. Paradoxically, the quiescent state is a function of softly resilient motion. We can only hold our bodies still through constant muscular tension and contraction. By constantly tensing and contracting the musculature, however, we effectively forfeit the condition of relaxation. We inhibit the natural flow of breath and the passage of energy through the body. By holding the body still, we transform the gelatinous nature of the body's tissues into a kind of armoring that is able to block out our awareness of the body's tactile sensations. The result of this physical holding and hardening is a mind filled with involuntary thoughts of attack and judgment, fear, desires, and fantasies. Clearly this is not the quiescent state of mind that we hope to create through the practice of meditation.

When applied appropriately to the process of meditation, stillness is a relative term at best. It is to be found between the two poles of an imposed immobility and a constant fidgeting. If we sit down to meditate and react to the appearance of every unpleasant sensation by moving or rearranging our body or even standing up and walking away altogether, our meditative inquiry cannot proceed very far. At the same time, if we impose an unnatural stillness on our sitting posture, we create the kinds of conditions outlined in the last paragraph. These too will seriously interfere with our progress. The introduction of subtle resilience into the posture of meditation allows us to avoid the pitfalls of these two extremes.

Resilience is a function of accepting and then yielding to the forces of nature that so affect and move through us. This may be the force of gravity, the sensations in the body, or the movement of the breath. Resilience is about flexibility and always involves surrendered motion. The leaf that dances on the wind is remarkably resilient. So too is the water of the ocean that allows the force of waves to move through it and constantly change its shape. The tallest trees and skyscrapers sway in the wind. If they didn't, they would break apart. Indeed, one of the greatest dangers to the tallest and most established trees is an unseasonal ice storm that leaves a layer of brittle ice covering the surface of the tree. If the tree is unable to continue its resilient swaying motion, it may snap apart.

Resilience is the quality that nurtures the conditions of alignment and relaxation and extends their presence over time. Alignment is not a static condition that we seek to create and then maintain. It is an ongoing process that may change from moment to moment. Relaxation is not a static gesture. It too is an ongoing process. The body continues to let go of tension and yield to the appearance of new areas of sensation that continually present themselves. In the posture of meditation the body is in constant, subtle motion. Without alignment there can be no relaxation, but without resilience there can be no relaxation either. Relaxation without resilience is a contradiction in terms. How can the body be relaxed, surrendering its weight constantly to the pull of gravity, and yet be tensing its musculature in an attempt to hold itself very still?

The final challenge for the meditator who has brought the body into a condition of alignment and then surrendered its weight to the pull of gravity is to invite the quality of softly resilient motion into the posture. Paying attention to the process of breath is one of the most direct ways through which we can contact the perpetual nature of subtle, resilient motion. The presence of breath belies the potentiality of stillness. Where there is breath, there is movement. If we hold our breath for any reason, we do so by holding our body still, and whenever we bring stillness into our body, we inhibit the breath. In that we breathe all the time, there is always going to be some accompanying movement even in the stillest of bodies. Furthermore, in an aligned and relaxed body this movement will not be limited to the area of the body around the organs of respiration proper (the chest and diaphragm), but can be experienced to extend throughout the whole body. Like a wave that moves without interference through a body of water, breath can be experienced to move through the entire length of an aligned and relaxed body. The force of breath invites the body to respond resiliently.

The action of breath is initiated through the involuntary contraction and relaxation of the diaphragm. The contraction of this powerful muscle creates a bellows effect that draws air into the lungs. Its relaxation encourages the oxidized waste to leave the body. With every contraction the belly can be seen to expand slightly; with every relaxation the belly becomes once again smaller. This amount of movement, so directly associated with the action of the diaphragm, exists in everyone (including the meditator who interprets the instruction to "sit still" to mean to sit with complete immobility).

In an aligned and relaxed body, however, the movement associated with breath need not be confined to this one small area of the body. Like ripples moving through a still pond into which a pebble has recently been dropped, the movement initiated by the involuntary action of the diaphragm can expand joint by joint through the entire body. As the diaphragm contracts, the belly and lower back expand slightly. In an aligned and relaxed body the force of this expansion can then be felt to move simultaneously up the torso through the top of the head and down through the pelvis and the legs. The amount of actual movement may be very small, but its existence is real. Ida Rolf once stated that in a completely relaxed and balanced body the motion of breath would generate subtle movement at every joint in the body and that this would include the sutures in the skull and the joints between the small bones in the feet!

Moving upward from the belly, the force of the belly's expansion can stimulate the chest to open. The chain reaction continues as the force from this opening is immediately transferred to the shoulders, down the arms, and into the hands, all of which can be felt to respond to the force of the breath and to move ever so slightly. Finally, the neck and head can be felt to bob on top of it all. With the exhalation the movement retraces its path. As the cycle of breath keeps continuing, the whole body can be felt to expand and contract in the manner of an amoeba. The movement down through the pelvis and the legs on the inhalation and back up into the naval on the exhalation is even subtler, but can still be distinctly felt. If this kind of resilient movement is unavailable, it is a sign that the body is still holding and bracing itself and has not yet relaxed as fully as it possibly can.

In addition to the movement of the breath, the sensational presence of the body itself is another strong force to which we are challenged to respond resiliently when assuming the posture of meditation. The significant letting go of tension that the posture of meditation activates powerfully loosens the lid on the long-contained cannister of the inner world of the body's tactile sensations. The body is revealed to be a dynamic process of vibratory phenomena, all of which can be distinctly felt. The sensations of the body can be felt to flow, shimmer, throb, and vibrate. Some of the sensations may be very pleasant, others extremely uncomfortable. In the face of the uncomfortable sensations it is all too common a reactive habit pattern to tense the body in an attempt to modify or completely conceal the discomfort. The movement of the sensations, however, kindles the force of purification that clears the mental and physical blockages keeping the states of awareness that are the goal of our meditation practice contained and unavailable. By not shutting down on the emerging sensations, whatever their nature, but remaining resiliently open to them, we allow the process of purification to continue, and our experience of meditation naturally deepens. By holding back on the powerful flows and surges of sensations that may occur, we lock ourselves into further patterns of tension, and the posture of meditation becomes even further elusive. Resiliently yielding to the breath and to the emerging awareness of the body's sensations are two of the most powerful ways in which we can ensure that our practice continues moving forward.

"Resilience is the function / Of the self forgotten," sings the seventeenth-century Chinese poet Han Shan Te Ch'ing in his poem "On Clear Mind."[1] This attitude is further reflected in the words of the Zen poet Ikkyu, "To harden into a Buddha is wrong." As we become increasingly familiar with the process and experience of resilience, we come to recognize how the superficial dimension of mind and identity, which our meditation practice is designed to pierce through, is itself a function of holding still. We cannot stay open to the senses and be lost in the internal monologue of the mind at the same time. Clear, unfiltered awareness of sensations, and by extension sounds and sights, can only truly occur in a body that is relaxed and resilient. If that body is challenged to respond resiliently to a motion that wishes to move through it and it declines, then that body reintroduces an element of tension and forfeits its relaxation. As the awareness of sensations recedes, the internal monologue of the mind reappears to take its place.

Most meditation practices, their superficial differences and goals notwithstanding, attempt to reveal our identification with the internal monologue of the mind as creating a fictive, or at least a highly limiting, sense of self. Indeed we all have the same name for this aspect of experience. We call the speaker of the monologue "I." By assuming that we are this "I," however, we block out all awareness of deeper, more expansive, and more wholesome awarenesses of identity.

By bringing resilience into the posture of meditation, the internal monologue begins naturally to subside. To confirm this statement, you will want to watch closely to see what happens when you begin to experience subtly resilient movement passing through the whole body as you sit in a balanced and relaxed posture. The movement may be so subtle that no one would be able to detect that you are not "sitting still." Observe the process of your mind carefully as you sit in this way. You may be surprised to find that the internal monologue does not have any stable ground on which to erect itself and project its dominant presence. This is especially true when the resilient movement is able to extend through the top of the head. At these moments the conventional sense of self begins to dissolve, and a more expanded sense of identity appears to fill the void left by the small self's vacancy.

_____

It may be easier to experience the breath moving resiliently through the whole body if you begin by lying down on your back on a soft surface. You may want to have a friend slowly read this section aloud to you as you lie down in this way. Rest your hands on your belly with the palms down, one on top of the other. Depending on the relative lengths of your arms and torso, one hand may completely cover the other or the fingers of one hand may barely be touching the other. Find the placement of your hands that is the most relaxed and comfortable for you.

Begin by simply observing the breath through bringing your awareness to the sensations of touch and movement. Do not feel that you need to change your pattern of breath in any way. If the pattern changes on its own, that's fine, but do not forcibly attempt to make it conform to an image of proper breathing that you may have. Resilience is a function of allowance, not of manipulation. Simply observe the breath as it is. You will begin to notice subtle movements in the body as you breathe. Perhaps the belly can be felt to rise and fall slightly with every breath. Perhaps there is movement in the chest but not in the belly. Observe where your body naturally moves in response to the breath and where it holds still. Again, do not try to change anything about your pattern of breath. Simply observe how it is for you right now. We become aware that we are breathing through observing the movements of the body, the sensations generated by these movements, or the sensations created by the passage of air around the nose and the mouth. Keep on patiently and passively watching until the awareness of your pattern of breath becomes quite clear to you.

On the next three breaths extend the exhalation as long as possible without causing undue strain. You may wish to visualize that a friend is pressing down on your ribcage with every exhalation, helping you to expel all the gaseous waste from your body. At the very bottom of the exhalation your friend releases the pressure, and the inhalation comes flooding back into the body. After you have taken these three breaths, allow your breath once again to resume whatever pattern is natural to it. Can you remember how your pattern of breath appeared just a few minutes ago prior to this imaginary intervention? Is it different now? How is it different? Keep allowing your breath to breathe you however it wants throughout this entire exercise. From one breath to the next its pattern may change on its own. If that happens, allow it, but do not feel that you need to change it in any way for any reason.

Now bring your attention back to your hands as they rest on your belly, one on top of the other. Surrender the weight of your hands and your belly to gravity, and feel the sensations of relaxation enter into this area of your body. As you continue to breathe in this relaxed condition, you will begin to notice that your hands are not still. The movements that you can detect may be very subtle, but they are very real. As your breath causes movement in your belly, your hands can be felt to move ever so slightly in response. Perhaps they move up toward the ceiling on the inhalation and back down on the exhalation. Perhaps they slide slightly away from each other on the inhalation and back together on the exhalation. There is no "correct" way for them to move. There is only your way. Stay as relaxed and resilient as possible, and you will discover how your hands move in response to the breath. Spend a number of breaths familiarizing yourself with this movement. Is it the same from breath to breath, or does it change?

Now forcibly cause your hands to stay still. Allow no movement in this part of your body, and observe what happens elsewhere. What happens to your breath? What happens to your sensations of relaxation? What happens in your mind? Holding still in any one small part of the body generates a subtle pattern of holding that spreads to affect the whole body. Resiliently releasing holding in any one small part of the body encourages release everywhere else as well. Once again allow your hands to begin to respond to the movement of the breath, and experience how different this feels.

Bring your awareness next to your elbows as they rest on the soft, supporting surface, and allow the sensations of relaxation to extend to this part of your body as well. If your hands and arms are truly relaxed, the movement that began in the hands can now be felt to extend down the length of your forearms and will cause your elbows to move ever so slightly. The elbows may move into the surface underneath you as you inhale and rise up slightly when you exhale. They may move into or away from the body on the inhalation and reverse their movement on the exhalation. Again, do not force your elbows to move in any particular way, but simply find the movement that is true for your body.

Notice how a chain reaction of subtle movement has begun to occur in your body as a result of the generative force of the breath. As the belly rises and falls, the hands respond. The movement in the hands is then transferred along the length of the forearms to the elbows. Once you have contacted this feeling of movement in the belly, the hands, and the elbows, forcibly stop it, and once again observe what occurs when you hold still in this way. Resilient movement is the norm in a relaxed and balanced body. If that movement does not naturally occur, you are unconsciously resisting somewhere in your body. Resistance is antithetical to relaxation. Release the tension and holding in your elbows, and allow them once again to respond to the movement of the breath.

Turn your attention now to your shoulders. A great many sources of movement come together in the shoulder girdle so it is not possible to predict what will actually occur as you consciously bring resilience into this part of your body. The shoulders may move in unison or quite differently one from the other. One may rise while the other falls. One may move outward while the other spirals up and toward the ceiling. Keep trusting your body to find the resilient pattern of movement that is completely natural for it. Also recognize that over time that pattern of movement may change quite spontaneously.

After you have contacted the resilient dance that occurs in the shoulder girdle in response to the movement of breath, consciously cause it to stop. Hold the shoulders very still, and observe what begins to occur. The difference in sensation may be quite dramatic. You may find that it is difficult to breathe or that the experience of stillness is accompanied by a sensation of tension or pain that does not feel natural. See how much more shallowly you breathe when you hold the body in this way. How does stillness affect your sense of self or the activities of your mind? What effect does releasing the tension and allowing resilient movement back into the shoulders have on you?

We often hold our heads very still. In fact, stillness in the head is a virtual prerequisite for the sustenance of the internal monologue of the mind. First bring relaxation to your neck and head, and then slowly begin allowing this part of your body to respond subtly to the movement that has been generated in your hands, arms, and shoulders by the breath. You may need to reposition your head slightly in order to find the placement that allows it to be most comfortably relaxed. Experiment with moving your head very slightly up or down so that the back of the head rests more squarely on the surface that you are lying on and the eyes are looking directly up toward the ceiling. Feel how the head can respond to the breath, how it can be felt to expand and contract ever so slightly. It may perhaps be felt to move up and back on the inhalation and down and forward on the exhalation. The movement pattern in the head may vary significantly from person to person, so keep experimenting until you find the movement that is appropriate for you. Once you have contacted the movement that is possible, once again contrast your experience by forcibly stopping that movement from occurring. By patiently contrasting the difference between holding and yielding, you will come to know the values of resilience and the ways in which your body can naturally allow it to occur.

The movements in the lower part of the body in response to the flow of breath are even more subtle, and yet they too can be distinctly felt. The actual movement may be experienced more on an energetic level as a kind of ebbing and flowing of sensation in the pelvis, the legs, and the feet. As you learn to tune into these subtler levels of movement, they may be experienced to extend to the upper body as well. In the manner of an amoeba, the whole body can be felt to pulse, to expand and contract with each inhalation and exhalation. You may experience a pronounced shift in consciousness as you contact this amoebalike pattern of movement. Watch what happens when one part of the body inadvertently begins to tense and becomes once again stiller. How does this affect the awareness of your body, the manifestation of your mind? Perhaps you begin to notice that your attention has wandered and a stream of involuntary thought has begun to occur. See if you can allow the internal monologue to continue, and simultaneously pass your awareness through your body to find where you have unconsciously re-created tension and resistance. You can learn a great deal about yourself simply by patiently observing the process of your body and mind through focusing on the possibility for resilient movement.

Once you have familiarized yourself with the possibility of a resilient pattern of breath that can move throughout the entire length of the body, you can bring what you have learned to your formal posture of meditation. Begin by bringing alignment and relaxation into your posture, and then slowly begin to add the element of resilience as you focus on every breath you take. You may wish to repeat the previous exercise in your sitting posture. Do not, however, expect that the body will respond and move in the same way as it did when you were lying down.

The resilient motion in the spine can become quite pronounced in the sitting posture. On the inhalation the entire spine can be felt to lengthen, and the spinal curves will flatten slightly. The head can be felt to rise up and back. The movement can even be felt to extend down into the sacrum. On the exhalation the spine settles down once again, and the spinal curves reestablish themselves.

Just as you did when you were lying down, you may want to contrast your experience of resilient movement by forcibly causing the spine to become still. Bring tension and holding in turn to the area of the sacrum and the lower back, the middle and upper back, the neck and the head. Notice how the reintroduction of stillness affects your breath, your experience of balance and relaxation, the meditative process itself. You may find that holding still in one or more of these areas feels very familiar to you. If this is so, make a special effort to bring resilience into this part of your spine.

Observe how your hands, arms, and shoulders can be felt to participate in the subtly resilient movement that your breath has initiated. As you sit in meditation, the entire body can be felt to be in motion. This motion may be so subtle that no one will be able to notice that you are not "sitting still." The motions that occur are completely natural and spontaneous motions. They cannot be induced or exaggerated to any benefit. Denying these motions, however, serves no benefit either and can be felt to seriously impede the process of meditation. Notice how relaxation is not possible unless resilience is present.

In addition to the breath there are two other major forces that can be resiliently responded to in the posture of meditation. The first of these is the force of gravity itself. Alignment, you will recall, is not a static state to be attained and then maintained. It is, rather, an ongoing process in which the small intrinsic muscles of the body are constantly making subtle and spontaneous adjustments to keep the body erect. Alignment is more of a dance than a pose. Stillness and holding can only inhibit the process of alignment and make the task of coming to balance much more difficult.

As you sit in the posture of meditation, exploring the possibilities for resilient movement, keep bringing your attention back to the experience of balance. Keep focusing on the feeling of the body as it continues to balance itself in as relaxed a condition as possible. Meditate on the relationship of the body to the gravitational field. Really feel this relationship, and see if you can continue to allow the most comfortable and relaxed condition of alignment to continue to manifest from moment to moment as the conditions of this relationship constantly shift.

You might like to review the movement exercises at the end of the chapter on alignment. In those exercises you experimented with gentle, swaying movements as you sat in the posture of meditation. Beginning with large, noticeable movements, you gradually reduced the range of motion until you came closer and closer to the imaginary vertical axis of alignment. At that point you were instructed to bring the movements to a stop as a way of pinpointing the exact location of the vertical axis. In practice, however, these slow, undulating, swaying movements never do come to a complete stop. By adding the elements of relaxation and resilience to the condition of alignment, the truly dynamic nature of the posture of meditation reveals itself. The body sways and moves around the vertical axis, but never comes to complete rest there. The motion is like a subtle jiggling or bobbing. The movements may be roughly circular or spiral in nature and are completely random. As the posture of meditation continues to refine itself, the movements become extremely subtle. They never, however, quit completely.

In addition to the breath and the force of gravity, the current of tactile sensations and the contents of the mind itself are constantly passing through the conduit of the body. If you hold back on this current for any reason, you will gradually create a condition of blockage that can only interfere with the posture of meditation. If you can learn to yield to this current, to respond to it resiliently, it will pass through you easily and comfortably without accumulating any residue or leaving any trace of its passage.

The holding and resistance that keep an imbalanced body erect also serve to keep the awareness of our deeper self contained. The complete storehouse of tactile sensations, feelings, emotions, and memories and thoughts that might be available to us becomes inaccessible. Bits and pieces may occasionally surface to remind us that much more is effectively buried and waiting to be unearthed, but the method by which we might excavate and uncover these deep contents is unclear.

The relaxation and release that the posture of meditation makes possible can bring these long-buried contents to the surface of awareness quite quickly. Often we may begin the process of meditation in a body that has little awareness of its tactile sensations. As we learn to relax through aligning the body, surrendering our weight, and then inviting the quality of resilience into our posture, this superficial awareness of numbness may rapidly begin to change. In its place a wide assortment of tactile sensations, pressures, and forces may suddenly appear. Some of the sensations may be quite neutral in tone. Others can become extremely pleasant. Still others may be very painful.

As you become increasingly aware of the tactile presence of the body, you will notice that the sensations that arise and pass away have a kind of motive force or current to them. Like almost everything else relating to the posture of meditation, they do not appear in a simple, static form, but are quite dynamic in their patterns of appearance and dissolution. Sometimes this rising and passing away occurs extraordinarily rapidly and on an extraordinarily minute scale as individual sensations appear to shimmer like tiny lights flickering on and off. At other times a large number of individual sensations mass together as a common force or presence. These sensations may appear like the force of water in a swiftly moving stream. Held rigidly, the body will resist the current of these sensations and cause them to accumulate and become jammed. In a condition of resilience, the body can yield to the force of these sensations and allow them to pass through in whatever way they need to.

As you become increasingly aware of these sensations, simply yield to them. Allow them to move through you in whatever way they wish. You may experience mild sensations of movement, like water passing through a hose, or you may experience powerful sensations of ebbing and flow as the sensations build to a heightened intensity and then dissipate. Sometimes, after long hours of sitting, the body may be experienced to shake or tremble as these sensational flows spontaneously bring themselves to resolution. Whenever you become aware of a sensation, simply accept it, allowing it to present itself in whatever form it wishes to take. You do not need to make the sensations stronger than they are. Nor do you need to hold back on their presence.

You may like to think of these emerging sensations as the manifestation of the unconscious contents of the body and mind. Ordinarily we are quite unaware of the tactile presence of the body. In other words, we are unconscious of it. Many somatic therapists are being drawn to the notion that the location for what we call the "unconscious" is to be found in the tissues of the body itself, not just in some corner of the brain. If this is so, then as we become increasingly conscious of sensations, we are literally bringing our unconscious to the surface of awareness where it can once again be liberated and included as part of the conscious sphere of our body and mind. The body is the repository of the unconscious only so long as we remain unconscious of the body.

Alternately, you may like to think of these emerging sensations as the manifestation of the life force. The life force wants to move through the body like a wave through water. If it becomes blocked, a sensation of pressure or pain will begin to form at the point of blockage. If you can learn to yield resiliently to this force, the body will spontaneously bring itself into a condition of alignment and relaxation and may experience an extraordinary condition of comfort, naturalness, and authenticity. Indeed, the ultimate cause of pain and suffering in the body can be directly attributed to the fearful resistance to allowing the life force to pass through the body without interference.

The comments that have been made about the flow of sensations in the body hold equally true for the passage of thoughts in the mind. Ordinarily we identify with the contents of our minds. As a thought emerges, we hold to it and claim it as our own. Like sensations, however, the force of the mind simply wishes to pass through us. If we respond by clinging to the contents or wishing to disavow and push them away, we create blockage that ultimately will manifest as holding and tension in the body and a dulling of awareness in the mind.

There are several different layers of thought that can be allowed to pass resiliently through the space of the mind and body just as wind moves through the branches of a tree. You do not need to hold on to any of them. The most superficial patterns of thought can be contacted as a force that wants to move through the space of the cranium and can be released through relaxing the area around the temples, the eyes, and the forehead. Deeper convictions of personal identity may be released and allowed to move through by consciously relaxing the area around the brain stem and the back of the throat. By holding and identifying with thoughts, you invite limitation into your experience and interfere with the passage of the life force just as effectively as if you were holding back on sensations.

Resilience implies movement. The movement, however, may be extremely subtle at times and difficult to detect. There may even be times during the movement when the sensations of the body or the contents of the mind begin to close down and become highly compressed. At times like this you may feel as though you are not able to respond resiliently and to allow the sensations to move through the body or the thoughts to dissipate through the mind. If this happens, do not force anything to occur, but simply accept this apparent moment of nonmovement as another phase in the process of resilience. Patiently accept and sink deeper into the experience. Trust the process of body and mind and the posture of meditation. Over time the deep blockage will yield, and the more familiar experience of flow and movement will reestablish itself. Never force. Accept everything. Hold to nothing. Resilience may imply movement, but it ultimately refers to complete acceptance of the natural manifestation of the life force. This force is deeply organic. It is our nature. We can contain it and miss its blessing, but we can never completely control it or predict the exact manner in which it will move.

NOTE
1. Ch'an Master Sheng-yen, *The Poetry of Enlightenment* (Elmhurst, New York: Dharma Drum Publications, 1987), p. 99.

5

Integration

THE POSTURE of meditation is a process in which the body initially aligns itself in the field of gravity, invites relaxation by surrendering its weight to the pull of that field, and then cultivates the conditions of alignment and relaxation through allowing the body to move and respond in subtly resilient patterns of motion. The posture of meditation is not a perfected condition which we aspire to attain and then maintain, but more like a work of art in continual progress and development. The three gestures of the posture of meditation—alignment, relaxation, and resilience—constantly influence and support one another. Alignment allows the body to relax. As the body relaxes, it becomes naturally more resilient. Over time a relaxed and resilient body will allow residues of tension and holding, at the levels of both the body and the mind, to come to the surface of awareness and resolve themselves. Through this resolution the alignment of the body will be affected in such a way that even greater relaxation and resilience may be possible. In this way the three gestures continually stimulate one another.

Just as the contents of the mind and body are observed during meditation to be in a condition of constant flux and change, so too will the posture of meditation itself constantly shift and refine itself. As we continue to gain access to ever deeper levels of awareness, more information (in the form of tactile sensations of the body and cognitive contents of the mind) will emerge that ultimately needs to be aligned, relaxed, and resiliently responded to. There may be times during your meditation when you come to a place in which the three postural gestures feel completely integrated. This state of integration does not signify that the posture has perfected or completed itself. A condition of perfection, with its implications of correctness and finality, is antithetical to the ongoing process of meditation. More often than not, moments of postural integration simply signify that you are on the threshold of dropping into a deeper layer of meditative awareness. Once this penetration begins to occur, additional tactile and cognitive data will begin to appear, and once again you will be challenged to process through this additional information through the gestures of alignment, relaxation, and resilience. In this way both the posture of meditation and the meditative awareness it promotes become increasingly refined over time.

Paradoxically, integration almost always signals transition and growth; it rarely denotes completion or stasis. Everything is in process, and nothing in the universe is capable of standing still. The desire to hold on to any object of experience, to maintain its status quo and render it impervious to change, is itself a cause of great suffering. Such a desire places us at odds with the universal law of change. This universal law applies as equally to our experience as human beings as it does to the appearance and dissolution of subatomic particles or the creation and destruction of entire worlds or planetary systems.

The phases in the process of change are reflected in the Hindu conception of the three forces of creation, preservation, and dissolution. These three forces take symbolic form in the Hindu trinity of deities: Brahma, Vishnu, and Shiva. Applied to the posture and process of meditation, this observation of universal change shows us that we must first work to create and establish the conditions of alignment, relaxation, and resilience. As we gradually let go of the physical and mental patterns of holding that interfere with the posture of meditation, a time naturally comes when the three gestures of this posture become integrated. The feeling tone of integration is extremely wholesome and joyous. Sitting in meditation, we suddenly feel as though we can sit forever, and indeed this feeling may sustain itself over a considerable period of time. Gradually, however, the integration itself allows the next deeper layer of psychophysical holding to come to the surface of awareness. When it does, the feeling of integration is dissolved as we are once again challenged to assimilate a great deal of emergent data. An alignment that is appropriate to the new emergent conditions of experience must now be created anew. This refined alignment allows deeper relaxation to occur, and our understanding of resilience will allow the relaxed state to expand and to be sustained. At some point an even further refined feeling of integration will appear. It will last as long as it is organically appropriate. Then it too will fade, and so the process continues over and over again.

In the beginning as we work with our posture, the initial creative gesture of finding and securing a condition of alignment may prove to be the most challenging of the three stages. Once we have familiarized ourselves over time with the posture and process of meditation, the stage of dissolution

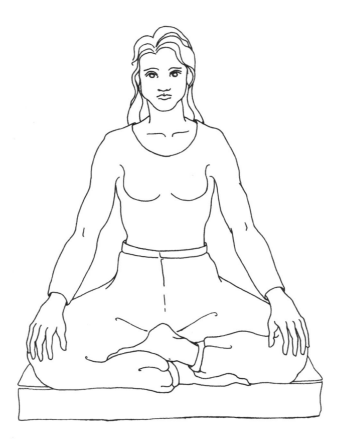

Balance is a function of alignment, relaxation, and resilience. When the body is balanced, nothing needs to be held on to or resisted. The force of gravity provides support for a balanced body, and the life force can pass freely through the body without interference.

may prove to be the most challenging. The posture of meditation is capable of dislodging deep psychophysical residues in the form of intensified emotional states in the mind and powerful energetic currents in the body. The manifestation of this residue is most potent during this final stage of dissolution. It is important to recognize that just as integration precedes dissolution, so too does dissolution precede entrance into a higher dimension of experience that ultimately will be integrated.

With this understanding it becomes easier to accept the periodic disorienting phases of the meditative process. During these moments the stability of alignment and the flowing quality of true relaxation may not be available or even appropriate. The ability to respond resiliently to the manifestation of this residue, however, is the most potent tool that can help you navigate these moments. Resilience in this context simply means allowance and acceptance. If powerful energetic surges are felt to build in the body, we can yield to them and allow them to pass through even if they temporarily move us into postural states that differ from our conventional understanding of alignment. If strong emotions and disturbing patterns of thought begin to emerge, we can yield to them as well. The key to working through these difficult periods is an attitude of trust and acceptance that permits the residue to come to the surface in as organic and natural a manner as possible. There is no need to stop it from emerging; nor is anything to be gained by indulging the process and attempting to make the emergent tactile sensations and patterns of thought even stronger or more prominent than they naturally are. Just to let them be is enough. Over time the body and mind will begin once again to settle, and alignment will once again reappear to bring a returned sense of stability into the practice.

Work to create the posture. Then trust in the process that it allows to emerge. Like a twig that falls into a river with a strong current, you will unfailingly be conveyed in the direction of the goal of your practice.

Part Two

Informal Practice

6

Moving through Life

As CHALLENGING as it may seem to bring alignment, relaxation, and resilience into our formal meditation posture, it may seem even more challenging to maintain these conditions and attitudes when we stand up and leave the relative haven of our meditation seat and begin moving out into the world. And yet this is exactly what we are asked to do.

Those of us who are householders may be able to find time for, at most, between half an hour and one or two hours of formal sitting practice a day. What, then, about the other twenty-two or twenty-three hours of the day? If we are sincere about progressing in our practice, we must recognize the importance of viewing the rest of our lives as "informal practice" and begin to bring the same calm and focused meditative awareness to all the activities of our lives, not just to the hours spent on our meditation cushions.

To some extent we are aided in this task by a kind of spill-over effect from our formal practice itself. Dedicated sitting practice inevitably yields results, and over time our lives do appear to become calmer, easier, and truer to our intentions, hopes, and highest purpose. It is unrealistic, however, to expect that our lives will be completely free from confusion, doubt, and ignorance simply because we sit in the formal posture of meditation for a short period of time every day. The posture of meditation can only be experienced *now,* and if we relinquish the embodiment of the posture as we go about our lives, we will be relinquishing the benefits and awarenesses that accompany that posture as well. Indeed, the fruits of meditative practice are a result of letting go of the habit patterns of the mind and the body that interfere with our clear awareness of this present moment.

Fortunately, we needn't leave the posture of meditation behind as we stand up from our formal sitting practice. Alignment, relaxation, and resilience can once again be our guides and companions as we move out into the world and interact with our families, colleagues, and friends. With this understanding we come to realize that meditation is something we do all the time, whether we are aware of this or not. By bringing alignment, relaxation, and resilience into our actions and movements through life, we begin to experience in our lives a benefit and change similar to what occurred when we first introduced these gestures into our formal sitting practice.

One of the main benefits of a formal sitting practice is that we take time out from the normal routines and pace of our lives and slow down considerably. We pay attention again to the primary events of our lives, phenomena that are completely remarkable and yet that we take almost completely for granted: the action of breath, the appearance and dissolution of bodily sensations, the drama of our minds, feelings, and emotions. Only by slowing down can we observe these phenomena, and only through observing and experiencing them closely can we learn from them and allow their patterns to change if we learn that change would be beneficial to us.

Relaxation is really the central key to the posture of meditation. Alignment can be viewed as a kind of precondition that makes relaxation possible, while resilience is the post-condition that allows relaxation to continue over time. If we begin to examine our lives with as much objectivity as possible and closely observe what we are actually doing from moment to moment, we are almost always struck by how unrelaxed we are. Many of us lead lives so filled with activities, duties, and responsibilities that we become over-whelmed and tend to shut down our awareness of bodily sensations so as not to feel the effects of the stress that inevitably builds as a result. The way we do this is to bring a great deal of tension into the body to enable us not to feel what is actually occurring. Others of us who are struggling to find a niche in life and a place to focus our energies may experience ourselves as underwhelmed. While this situation brings with it a different quality of pain and unsatisfactoriness, the preferred remedy for dealing with this pain is exactly the same as the one used for dealing with stress: by bringing tension into the body and turning our awareness away from the lived truth of this very moment we shield ourselves from having to feel what is actually going on in our lives. While these strategies may have a certain amount of short-term effectiveness, over time they can generate a great residue of tension, and real relaxation becomes very elusive indeed.

What would happen, however, if we were simply to slow down and to begin to pay more attention to what we were actually doing in any given moment? Driving a car, cooking a meal, working in an office or factory, exercising, sitting at a computer, talking with our friends and family, mowing the lawn, playing with our children: every occasion in life presents an opportunity to explore the posture of meditation. By bringing alignment, relaxation, and resilience into all activities of our lives, we effectively transform them into situations capable of revealing to us the highest insights and understandings.

The first thing that you may notice as you begin to observe your movements through life is how much of the time you spend lost in the inner monologue of your mind. If you pay close attention, you will also come to recognize that when your internal voice is particularly active you have very little conscious awareness of anything else that is occurring: the sensations in your body, the sounds, sights, smells, and tastes that surround and penetrate you. You will further come to realize that the unbridled momentum of the inner monologue is itself dependent on a specific bodily posture or attitude. You may only be able to come to recognize this retrospectively, because when you are lost in your mind, you really are unaware of the rest of sensory reality. (In truth, most of the time when our inner monologue is particularly active we have little awareness of the monologue as well.) In any case, as you become more sensitive and able to monitor what is actually transpiring, you will become aware that the internal monologue of the mind is dependent on a condition of explicit holding and tension in the body. This pattern of holding is almost completely opposite from the posture of meditation. The alignment of the body is compromised. There is no real relaxation and very little resilience.

Unfortunately, it is some variation or other on this pattern of holding that passes as normal in the modern world. Is it any surprise, then, that the kinds of conscious states that deep meditation practice allows us to contact and experience are rare occurrences for most of us? What passes as normal in the world at large is a kind of awakened sleep state. Much like when we walk in our sleep, we manage not to bump into things, but have little real awareness about what is actually transpiring around us. By not actively bringing the posture of meditation into our activities in life, we are simply supporting the prevailing belief that there is something taboo about the nature of human experience that manifests naturally in an aligned, relaxed, and resilient condition of embodiment.

We bring alignment into our lives by paying attention to how the energy field of our body relates to the gravitational field of the earth. The same primary principles of verticality that governed our ability to bring the body to alignment in the formal sitting posture allow us to maintain that alignment as we move through life. If the body can efficiently organize itself around a predominantly vertical axis in any of its activities, then the field of gravity can reinforce and support the energy field of the body.

The application of alignment is most apparent in activities such as standing, walking, or sitting. Much like the formal sitting posture, these activities allow you to organize the mass of your body around a predominantly vertical spine. How do we apply the underlying principles of alignment, however, to all the other movements we can make in which the spine is not so vertical? The simplest answer to this question comes through the recognition that alignment allows us to do things in the simplest, most efficient manner possible. When we perform any movement efficiently we are applying the principles of alignment.

These other movements, with the exception of lying down, are all variations on the action of bending. We lean forward or to the side. We bend over to pick something up or to position ourselves to play a game. Bending motions are inherently unstable because they demand that a certain amount of tension be introduced into the relationship between the energy field of the body and the gravitational field of the earth. They are transitional postures, and we can never rest comfortably in a bent position for very long. When you bend, you temporarily relinquish the verticality of the spine and the support of gravity. Even when you bend, however, you can continue to play with balance. Parts of the body will move in front of the imaginary vertical axis through which gravity flows; others will move behind this axis in compensation. Through the coordinated orchestration of these compensating movements the overall condition of balance can be maintained. By consciously playing with balance in whatever action you are performing, you are supporting the embodiment of alignment. Remaining aware of your condition of balance allows you to enter into a bending posture and then return back into a more vertically aligned posture without unconsciously accumulating any unnecessary tension.

Pay attention to alignment as much as possible in whatever you're doing. Pay attention to the feeling tones and sensations that are generated throughout the body as you focus in this way. Notice how different these sensations are when alignment is not present. Notice how alignment directly affects your state of awareness. Watch what happens to your awareness when you forfeit your alignment. Pay attention as you stand up from your meditation seat, as you walk through your house, as you bend to pick up a magazine, as you prepare and eat your meals (and clean the kitchen afterward), as you take a shower, as you drive to work, as you interact with friends, fellow workers, your children, your parents, your lover.

Once you have familiarized yourself with the feeling tones and sensations of alignment you will be able to begin to monitor yourself, and you will be able to recognize instantly if you are encouraging alignment or temporarily forgetting about it. It is very important to remind yourself that alignment is a lived experience that generates specific awarenesses, sensations, and feeling tones. It is not just an abstract set of spatial coordinates applied to the structure of the body. Alignment is the ongoing play and dance of balance. Let these very alive feeling states guide your body ever closer toward a condition of real structural alignment. When your body becomes aligned with the directional flow of gravity, these feeling states will be present. In whatever action you perform, if your body remains comfortably balanced, these feeling states will also appear. If you stand in front of a mirror and try to force your body into what appears to be an ideal vertical alignment, you will almost certainly generate tension and holding that will not permit the feeling states of alignment to emerge. Every body is different. Find your own way to alignment. There is no such thing as an ideal template to which you must force your body to conform. There are only feelings, sensations, and awareness. Let them continue to be your primary guide. Find the alignment that is appropriate to your body at this moment, recognizing that it may continue to change and become more refined in the next moment. Imagine that the world in which we live is a huge swimming pool filled with the most buoyant salt water, and alignment allows us to float. Keep floating and playing in this wonderful pool of gravity. How can you bring alignment and balance into this very moment? How does that affect your experience of this moment? Can you continue to bring alignment and balance into this next moment? Apply the exercises at the end of the chapter on alignment not just to your formal sitting posture, but to your standing, walking, and moving about.

As you move through the successive activities of your day, allow more and more relaxation to enter into your body. Relaxation means to do whatever you are doing in the easiest way possible. When Chuang Tzu stated that "easy is right," he was encouraging us to bring as much relaxation as possible into our lives. Life becomes easier when we make the enormous force of gravity our ally rather than our adversary. It is easier to align our bodies with the directional flow of gravity and then relax by surrendering our weight to gravity than it is to brace ourselves constantly against gravity. Relaxation means to let go of unnecessary tension. How much tension can you let go of as you take a leisurely walk? Can your arms hang loosely from your shoulders, or do you feel that you need to hold them up to secure your balance? Can your belly hang comfortably and easily as you breathe and move, or do you unconsciously hold it in? In order to relax you need to develop trust in the field of gravity as your ally. The feeling states of alignment help you to develop this trust, and your experimentation with relaxation will further it significantly. Familiarize yourself with the deeply wholesome feeling states of relaxation. They are your birthright.

As you continue slowly to walk, monitor the sensations in your body and the activity in your mind. The sensations of relaxation have a distinct and recognizable quality to them. They feel softly vibrant and nourishing. As soon as tension enters back into a part of the body the sensations begin to change. The sense of loosely flowing vibrancy gives way to numbness or tightening. The sensations no longer feel healing, but feel as though they need to be healed. A relaxed mind is comfortably alert, able to monitor the different sensory data with which the body is constantly challenged to interact. In a tense body the mind loses its mirrorlike quality, its sense of clarity and alertness. Even though the eyes are open, it may not really see what is in front of it. Sounds may pass by unnoticed. Sensations and feeling states may be blocked out or ignored. In a tense body the mind may be clouded with a layer of involuntary thoughts that have little application to the current situation in which you find yourself. Making matters worse, we often identify ourselves with this layer of thoughts and forget about the depths of being that lie beyond them.

As you continue to experiment and familiarize yourself with alignment and relaxation, you will learn to distinguish between the feeling states of alignment and misalignment, relaxation and tension. The more familiar you become with these different sensations and feeling states, the easier it will be for you to maintain the process of aligning and relaxing the body and mind. Tension reenters the body and mind when you react with clinging or aversion to any bit of sensory data with which you interact: a sight, a sound, a bodily sensation, even a thought or memory. As soon as this reaction occurs, the feeling tone of relaxation is lost and is replaced by the growing feeling tone associated with tension. As you learn to monitor your sensations, it becomes much easier to catch yourself when a reaction has occurred and to let go of whatever tension has developed as a result. In this way you can continue to let go of tension and invite relaxation, and its attendant benefits, into your posture as much as possible.

From moment to moment as you move through life relaxation is possible. The habit pattern of reaction is so subtle and ingrained, however, that you will continually be challenged to remember to relax, to let go of tension, to learn how to do things as easily as possible. The way you eat your food, drive a car, bathe yourself, wash the dishes: there are no activities in life to which the action of relaxation cannot be appropriately applied. Inevitably you will find that it is easier to bring relaxation into some situations than into others. Relaxation generally involves a noticeable slowing down. You may find, for example, that you need to slow your normal pace considerably if you wish to walk in a truly relaxed way. Learning to do things differently always brings challenges. As you walk more slowly down a familiar city street, you may experience yourself and the neighborhood in quite a different way. Can you stay open to this new awareness? Do you feel more vulnerable when you relax in this way? Do you feel stronger? Is it okay to feel this vulnerability or strength? By applying the posture of meditation to your movements through life, you will inevitably begin to experience a profound transformation in your body and mind. Can you accept this transformation? Can you accept who and what you become when you move in this way? Sometimes your conventional pattern of holding, even though it is painful, has an appeal due to the comfort of its familiarity. Can you shift your goal as you walk from reaching your destination as quickly as possible to relaxing into the experience of the present moment as you move along your path?

Surrendering your weight to the pull of gravity does not just diminish and transform the sensations of physical tension. Inevitably the self-created masks or personae through which we interact with the world begin to soften and fall away as well. Commitment to the posture of meditation will force you to let go of the unconscious reliance on different masks or ways of posing in the world. It will allow you instead to meet and become familiar with a deeper, more authentic sense of self, one that does not need to rely on artificial poses and projections of self-image. This deeper self may simultaneously feel completely natural and yet empty of specific definition. It too is marked by a definite and recognizable feeling state. Relaxation leads you directly to this deeper self. Once you have contacted it, relaxation continues to nurture and support it. This deeper self may feel radically different from your conventionally egoic sense of self. It may feel more like empty space than the solidified entity that the ego would like to convince you is your true nature. Can you allow this deeper self to continue over time, or do you feel an almost unconscious urge to cover it over and resurrect your more recognizable and conventional sense of self? To reassert your more familiar sense of self, you must bring tension back into your body. We all want relaxation. How relaxed are you willing to let yourself be? If your conventional awareness of self begins to dissolve through relaxation, can you simply accept the new condition and allow the relaxation to continue? What happens when this transformation occurs on your sitting cushion? What happens when it occurs while you're walking down a busy city street? What happens when it occurs when you are walking alone along a remote mountain trail? Are you able to allow this emerging transformation to continue if you are at a social gathering?

Resilience completes the posture. A relaxed body does not artificially hold itself still. Like a small child, it does not need to resist the impulse to move responsively. As a body continues to become more relaxed, it naturally becomes more resilient. Its movements become more streamlined, coordinated, and graceful. Resilience extends relaxation over time. With every breath you take, the body can respond resiliently. With every movement you perform, the body can respond resiliently. True resilience of movement involves the entire body acting as a coordinated unit of interdependent parts. The slightest movement in any one part of the body can spread throughout the entire body. A sudden movement in the head or the shoulders can be transferred joint by joint through the entire body and ultimately be felt in the feet. Like a wave that laps against a rock and then returns back toward the ocean from which it came, the movement may not stop there. It may instead begin to move back up the body, arriving back at the area where the initial movement originated. By remaining open to the possibility of resilience, the body can stay in perpetual, subtle motion. Paradoxically, this motion will not exhaust the body, but will keep it refreshed and vibrant. To hold the body artificially still is exhausting. Great grace enters effortlessly into the actions of a person who can move resiliently.

Riding in a car presents a wonderful opportunity to practice and explore resilience. Ordinarily we hold ourselves very still as we sit in or drive a car. We brace ourselves against the bumps of the road and the motion of the car. If we relax and allow our bodies to respond resiliently to the ride, however, our experience will be quite different. The body rocks randomly up and down and from side to side. The head, which is ordinarily held very still in a car, bobs and jiggles atop it all. Play with this resilient motion the next time you ride in a car. Then hold your body very still in contrast and observe how different this feels. Can you relax your arms and your hands as you hold on to the steering wheel? Does placing a small cushion behind your back improve your alignment?

Sitting at a desk, you may need to reach forward to grasp an object. Do you reach forward only with your arm, keeping the rest of your body completely still and braced? Or can your entire body, even down to your ankles, participate in the simple action of reaching forward? Observe how much less tension is felt to exist if your entire body can participate in a coordinated and resilient manner. Observe how much more alert and clear your mind is if you reach forward in this way.

Alignment, relaxation, and resilience can be experienced in everything we do. The effect of their coordinated interaction is particularly noticeable in the action of the breath. When the body is aligned, relaxed, and resilient, the breath is naturally smooth and long. Inhalations and exhalations flow smoothly one into the other. The pacing of the breath is regular and even. Over time it may begin to feel as though the breath were moving through the entire length of the body, cleansing the sensations of the body of any residual tension through its movement. If this cleansing and wholesome quality of breath is absent, you can be certain that the posture of meditation has been somehow compromised. Any holding in the body will interfere with the free and natural movement of the breath. As we release unnecessary holding through embracing the posture of meditation, the breath naturally assumes a pattern of fullness, length, and regularity. Combining an awareness of breath with an awareness of alignment, relaxation, and resilience can create a powerful meditative base with which to walk through life.

Alignment, relaxation, and resilience are ultimately capable of transforming consciousness itself. The effects of holding in the body are not just limited to the creation of painful physical sensation and restriction of the free flow of the breath. They also create holding and tension in the mind. They fuel the internal monologue and directly support the fearful and limited view of the world that the monologue would like to convince us is an accurate reflection of reality. As the monologue gains a firmer foothold in our consciousness, the body tightens even more.

As you learn more and more to bring the posture of meditation into the activities of your life, the meditative states and goals that your formal sitting practice is designed to lead you to may begin to become more commonplace. Gradually you will come to recognize that the effect of embodying the three primary gestures of the posture of meditation is not just limited to an improvement of the mechanical function of the body. As tension and holding are released from the body, the hard edges of mental tension that manifest in the limited ways in which we view ourselves and the world begin to soften as well. It cannot be otherwise, for just as holding and tension in the body create holding and tension in the mind, so also does the release of physical holding and tension release mental restrictions, contractions, and limitations as well. This relationship will become particularly apparent over time as your ability to embody the posture of meditation becomes increasingly refined. As it does, you will be challenged to let go of many of the limiting beliefs and perceptions with which you may have formally identified yourself. It is simply not possible to enjoy the increased sense of physical well-being and the improvement of physical function generated through the posture of meditation while simultaneously holding on to these limiting beliefs and perceptions. As this refinement occurs you will also begin to realize that the meditative states of awareness that are becoming increasingly common are not exotic or special in any way, but are simply the natural state of a person who is aligned, relaxed, and resilient. Instead of relying on the many beautiful and inspiring descriptions of this natural state that can be found in spiritual literature, trust more and more in the posture, and discover this state for yourself.

As with any skill the posture of meditation requires patient practice if we hope to become proficient in its application. This is what the Buddha meant when he urged his followers to work out their own salvation with diligence. By diligently and patiently bringing as much attention as possible to alignment, relaxation, and resilience in everything we do, we become increasingly skilled in the art of living and dying. Practice patiently, but never with tension. You cannot force the posture of meditation into existence. You can only allow it to emerge as you keep letting go of whatever restrictions . to its manifestation are revealed through your patient inquiry. Ten thousand times a day the posture will burst into awareness. Ten thousand times a day it will become lost again as the former habit patterns of your body and mind reestablish themselves. Over time, however, the long hours of practice begin to pay off, and your former habit patterns begin to weaken and dissolve. New ones will now emerge to fill their place, and these new patterns will be based on the principles of body and mind that the posture of meditation directly supports. And when such a transformation begins to embody itself in the tissues and patterns of your body and mind, you will realize that you have moved much closer to attaining the goal of whatever form of meditation practice you have been fortunate to have brought into your life.

Afterword

ALIGNMENT, relaxation, and resilience are for everybody. Unlike individual sports, which tend to favor certain body shapes and sizes over others, the posture of meditation is available to everyone. It does not matter whether you are tall or short, heavyset or slender. It does not matter how flexible you are. By conscientiously exploring and applying the principles of the posture of meditation, you will gradually become adept in bringing alignment, relaxation, and resilience into your life. There is no ultimately perfect posture that you need to strive to embody. There is only the posture that is appropriate for your particular body, and your body is unlike anybody else's. The first taste of alignment, relaxation, and resilience will significantly transform your posture and experience. Subsequent tastes will refine that experience, adding subtle dimensions and nuances of sensation that you may have never known about. The posture of meditation is a process, not a goal. The application of the three primary gestures will allow you to experience the insights that are appropriate to your development at this particular moment in time. Benefits begin immediately and continue over time.

The principles and exercises in this book will allow you to

let go of the patterns of holding and tension that keep the posture of meditation hidden. They will work for everybody, regardless of an individual's physical conditioning and state of tension. The process of meditation allows us to unravel whatever physical and psychic knots we may have accumulated over time. Our job is to engage the process and to allow it to affect and transform us. We do not get gold stars after our name if we can manifest the posture of meditation quickly and suddenly. Nor is it a mark of judgment against us if the posture manifests only slowly over time. The posture allows us to contact the truth of our condition, whatever that condition may be. By contacting the truth of our condition, the unraveling process has no choice but to begin.

If you come to a point of impasse in your exploration of alignment, relaxation, and resilience, you may choose to keep patiently allowing the posture to resolve the blockage or you may choose to seek out the services of a professional from within the field of somatic (that is, body-oriented) education. Depending on the nature of the impasse, you may find help through a Rolfer, an acupuncturist, a chiropractor, a Feldenkrais or Alexander practitioner, or a dance therapist. The field of somatic therapy is extremely diverse, and a wide range of techniques, each focusing on a different aspect of embodiment, is to be found in the marketplace. Some techniques focus on the more purely mechanical condition of the body; others view the physical condition primarily as a metaphor through which to define and resolve emotional or attitudinal blockages. If you choose to explore this broad field as an adjunct to your meditation practice, it is advised that you open yourself fully to the teachings of the technique you have chosen, but never lose sight of the reason you sought assistance from the somatic practitioner in the first place. Many somatic therapists view the increase in pleasurable sensation, or the resolution of the physical blockage, as the ultimate goal of the work. To a student of meditation, however, the relief or release of tension is only significant to the degree that it helps you gain insight into the meditative states of awareness to which your formal practice is leading you. Many students of meditation explore the field of somatic education as an adjunct to their practice. Perhaps in a thousand years' time, when an historian of spiritual practices looks back on our era, the exploration of somatic practices will appear to be an introductory phase in the process of meditative inquiry. Explore these practices if necessary, but never lose sight of the guiding principles of alignment, relaxation, and resilience and their ability to lead you ever closer to your intended goal.

Finally, anybody wishing to correspond with the author or to receive information about workshops and retreats based on the principles presented in this book may do so by contacting the Institute for Embodiment Training, RR 2, Cobble Hill, B.C., VOR ILO, Canada.